PRIVATIZATION

The Proceedings of a Conference

Hosted by the
National Center for Policy Analysis
and the
Adam Smith Institute

Edited by
John C. Goodman

To David Denholm
with warm regards
John C. Goodman

ISBN 0-943802–13-X

Table of Contents

Introduction

On October 12, 1984 a conference was held in Washington. To my knowledge no conference like it had ever been held before.

The conference was attended by the leaders from the major public policy research institutes, by academics and researchers interested in policy issues, and by individuals who work in the Washington bureaucracy. The theme of the conference was: How Ideas Cause Change.

On the surface, it might not seem unusual for representatives from think tanks to get together to discuss how ideas influence public policy. After all, that is what think tanks are supposed to be all about. And yet, this conference was unusual. It is instructive to consider why.

Throughout history, intellectuals have always believed that ideas cause change. We even can trace major political events back to the originators of the ideas that seemed to inspire these events. Yet why is it that some ideas cause change and not others? And when an idea does lead to change, exactly how does it do so?

Historically, our understanding of how this works has always been general and vague. For example, the following explanation of the process was once given to me by a professor of philosophy: Philosophers, he said, are the originators of all new great ideas. From the philosophers ideas flow to the other academic disciplines and then into books. From books they flow to newspaper editors and editorial writers; from newspaper editorials they flow to the comic strip writers; and from the comic strips they flow to the general public.

This explanation, though quaint, leaves us in the position of having to wait (Lord knows how long) until another brilliant philosopher emerges before we can have change. Even then, we have no idea what the new ideas will be or what subsequent changes will be forthcoming.

But suppose there is a different way. Suppose there is a way of generating ideas that by their very nature are destined to change public policy. And suppose there is a way of systematically generating a whole series of ideas destined not just to change a single policy, but the whole direction of government itself. If this were possible, it would be enormously important to the public policy community. The process also would be crucially important to individual think tanks. Yet, strange as it may seem, prior to 1980 this line of thinking had never been seriously pursued.

Three events changed all this. Each was essential. If any of these three events had failed to occur, this conference would never have been held.

Event Number One. During the late 1960s and throughout the 1970s a revolution was occurring in political science. Called "public choice theory," "economic theory of regulation," or the "new political science," this revolution consisted of creating rigorous mathematical models of political systems and attempting to explain in a scientific way how governments work. Antony Downs, William Riker, James Buchanan, Gordon Tullock and George Stigler were some of the early contributors to this movement. They all shared the common practice of using analytical tools developed by economists to explain political phenomena.

For any intellectual who believed in freedom and free enterprise, the 1970s was an exciting time to be alive. The academic landscape was changing rapidly. Before this time the old academic order was permeated with the "benevolent" view of government. Even the economics textbooks routinely portrayed government as an institution which intervened in private affairs to increase social welfare and make people better off. It is not clear why this view was widely held. Even a casual glance at governments around the world and even a minimal knowledge of history should be enough to establish that at most times and in most places government is the primary cause of great human misery. It is strange that the benevolent view of government was given any credence at all, but it was.

I can recall as a doctoral student at Columbia University during those years, I was trying to explain how regulatory agencies set prices. Sam Peltzman was independently pursuing the same line of thought at UCLA. We both reached the same conclusion: Government regulators consistently will make bad choices in setting prices. And they do so not because they are corrupt or because they lack the will to do the right thing, but because they have no choice.

The key to the new political science was the realization that competition among politicians and political parties for votes is analogous to competition among business firms for sales dollars. In the political competition, the desire for victory leads politicians to adopt winning policies (called "equilibrium" policies) whether or not they are good policies. In fact, the equilibrium policies almost never will be good policies. Put another way, decision-making through the political process is inherently defective because the decision-makers are inevitably and inexorably driven by the process of political competition to make bad policy decisions.

The new political science threatened the very foundations of contemporary liberal thought. What it said was: What liberals expect from government they systematically will be denied. No wonder that the new theory was opposed not only by traditional political scientists but also by many economists. Fortunately, the opposition was weak and ineffective and destined to subside.

As exciting and revolutionary as the new political theory was, it left many unanswered questions. For example, almost all of the theoretical models were static, rather than dynamic, and had little to say about why political changes occur over time. In addition, they all seemed to accept a pervasive determinism, suggesting that individual efforts to change things were futile. More importantly, the political models had no room for the role of ideas.

Event Number Two. For this one we can thank Mother Nature. In December, 1976, a snow storm hit New York City, and it took a week for the city's sanitation department to clear the streets. Reeling from angry protests on the part of the citizenry, Mayor Lindsay assigned one of his aides, E.S.Savas, the task of finding out why the Sanitation Department could not remove the snow from New York City streets in a timely and efficient way.

Needless to say, Savas found that the Department of Sanitation was riddled with waste and inefficiency and was poorly managed. But he did not stop there. Savas was no ordinary bureaucrat. He was a well-trained economist who knew how to gather statistics and analyze them.He knew how to do research and how to present his findings in an impeccable, scholarly way.

What Savas did was rigorously analyze and compare the performance of the city's Department of Sanitation with the performance of private refuse collectors. What he found was that the quality of New York City garbage collection could be greatly improved and that its cost could be cut in half by contracting out the entire enterprise to private firms.

Savas possessed one other skill not commonly found in the ranks of the bureaucracy or in academia. He had natural public relations skills—skills that served him well in publicly televised debates with the head of the Sanitation Department and in other forums.

Savas did not get all of the changes he wanted, but he did get some. More changes followed. One can only wonder what went through his mind at the time. It must have been a heady experience considering his background. Coming from the academic world, Savas knew that studies by academics rarely produce change. Having worked in the New York City bureaucracy he also knew change rarely was produced by going through normal bureaucratic channels.

But now, two important thoughts must have occurred to him. First, through his collecting of facts and making them public—on television, on radio and through the newspapers—the bureaucracy reacted and changed its ways of doing things. Second, these changes had been achieved while he was an employee of New York City government. He had used the resources of government to help shrink the size of government, or at least slow its rate of increase. He had started the U.S.privatization movement.

If it could work for refuse collection, what about street cleaning, bus operations, and dozens of other services provided by government? Later, as Undersecretary at the Department of Housing and Urban Development (HUD), he would use the grant-making powers of the department again to marshall the resources of government to help reduce its size. He funded a number of very expensive research projects, resulting in irrefutable evidence of the benefits of privatization in virtually every aspect of city government.

Fifteen years after a freak snow storm hit New York City, Savas would address a group of mayors in the Pacific Northwest. The question there was not: Should we privatize? Instead the question was: How do we do it? At the local level, the intellectual battle had been won.

By all accounts, one of the most important things Savas did while at HUD was organize an international seminar on privatization. In attendance was Madsen Pirie, president of the Adam Smith Institute in London.

Event Number Three. In the early 1980s Madsen Pirie was a brilliant young philosopher who was frustrated. After a brief stint at Hillsdale College in Michigan and then at the Heritage Foundation in Washington, he moved to London in the mid-1970s with a modest ambition: To bring freedom and free enterprise to England.

Britain represented socialism at its worst. In the early 1950s Britain had one of the highest standards of living in all of Europe. By the late 1970s, however, the ravages of socialism had left it with one of the lowest standards of living in all of Europe. Everyone knew something had to be done. No one knew how.

Enter Margaret Thatcher. Her 1979 election as Prime Minister brought with it the promise of great hope. Perhaps more than anyone else in British politics, Mrs.Thatcher was firmly and ideologically committed to the ideals and institutions of a free market economy. Early in her administration changes had been hoped for; unfortunately none were forthcoming.

In what Pirie later would call "Strategy I," Margaret Thatcher attempted to use all of the traditional conservative remedies for big government: abolish unnecessary programs, eliminate waste, impose budget limits on particular programs, and cut overall spending. None of these worked.

Then came "Strategy II": privatization. It was a strategy which would allow Margaret Thatcher to succeed where so many other conservative leaders in other countries had failed. It was a strategy which would make Britain a privatization showcase for the world. The Adam Smith Institute, under the direction of Madsen Pirie, can claim much of the credit for that.

Briefly, the secret of successful privatization is as follows: The public choice theorists were right. Once the issues are defined and the political coalitions are formed, the political system tends to move to a political equilibrium. There is not much that any political leader can do to move very far away from this equilibrium, unless the terms of the political debate are changed. But, the terms of the debate *can* be changed. They can be changed by introducing a new, previously unconsidered issue. For example, rather than argue about the level of spending for a program, why not simply propose that it be moved to the private sector, as had E.S.Savas. Once the new proposal is taken seriously, the old equilibrium begins to shatter as old coalitions dissolve and new ones are formed based upon new perceptions of self-interest.

Of course, in making the new proposal one wants to cloak it in such a way that it has great appeal to powerful interest groups. People and groups that have the power to block change must discover that the change is in their self-interest. Herein lies the beauty of privatization. What E.S.Savas discovered can be generalized. Privatization, always and everywhere, has the potential to save government money. Moreover, from this savings policy-makers have ready access to a new source of cash, some of which can be used to create benefits to elicit support from potential opponents. Put crudely, privatization in principle always produces sufficient savings to "buy off" the potential opponents of privatization.

That is how the British have achieved unprecedented privatization; every successful privatization attempt has followed this format.

In the spring of 1983, the National Center for Policy Analysis asked Madsen Pirie to write a book describing the 22 techniques that Margaret Thatcher has used to achieve successful privatization in Britain. Although the focus of the book was on Britain, and although all of the practical illustrations of privatization came from Britain, the book actually was a theoretical work, world-wide in scope and application.

It was an unprecedented contribution to political theory. It was the first book ever published which described how to systematically generate ideas that cause change. The book, *Dismantling the State: The Theory and Practice of Privatization* is the companion book to this volume, *Privatization.*

In the fall of 1984, the NCPA held a conference to introduce Pirie's book (then only in manuscript form) to the public policy community in the U.S. What follows are the proceedings of that conference.

As the reader will gather from these proceedings, events in one country often reinforce similar events in another. The process is helped along by individuals and institutes exchanging ideas and techniques.

In the late 1970s Robert Poole, president of the Reason Foundation, wrote a book called *Cutting Back City Hall.* The book described case studies of successful privatization at the local level in the United States. It became a valuable resource for Madsen Pirie and Eamonn Butler at the Adam Smith Institute in London. By pointing to successful examples of privatization in the U.S., Pirie and Butler were able to strengthen the argument for privatization in Britain.

In the early 1980s, Pirie attended the privatization seminar organized by E.S.Savas in Washington and told the American audience about privatization success stories in Britain. This no doubt helped spur a major research effort, funded at Savas' urging, on privatization in the U.S., and later made possible the establishment of the privatization data bank established at the Reason Foundation. The chain of events had come full circle.

At the local level in the U.S., a privatization revolution is underway. Details of this revolution are contained in "Privatization in the U.S.: Cities and Counties," included as an appendix to this volume. It is a revolution which has been underway for almost two decades.

At the federal level, things have been very different. At the time of this writing, the Reagan Administration has made some modest progress in spurring privatization in transportation at the local level through the funding policies of the Department of Transportation. But despite a prolonged and determined effort, the Administration still has been unable to sell Conrail.

At the federal level there has been no major privatization achievement. This is strange, because since 1980, and primarily following the lead of Britain, privatization has become a worldwide phenomenon. Governments around the world are selling off assets—state-owned airlines, banks, steel mills, etc. By some accounts the developing countries are making greater headway than the developed countries. But far from being a leader in the movement, Washington has largely by-passed the privatization revolution. Despite the ideological commitment to freedom and free enterprise, the Reagan Administration, until recently, has shown little interest in the subject. One of the purposes of this conference was to help remedy that.

Here again, it is interesting to see how the movement of people and ideas across the Atlantic can help to propel a movement. Before founding the Adam Smith Institute in London, Madsen Pirie and Eamonn Butler worked at the Heritage Foundation in Washington. Under the leadership of Edwin Feulner, the Heritage Foundation was quickly evolving into the bellwether institute for conservative thought in America. It was at Heritage that Pirie and Butler learned about the mechanics of running a public policy institute. They learned from the very best.

In setting up the Adam Smith Institute, they were joined by a third individual: Eamonn's brother, Stuart. Stuart Butler left the Heritage Foundation and moved to London to help start the new institute. Later, he returned to the Heritage Foundation. Each of these moves was important because they represented an idea change. More than any other single individual, Stuart Butler has been primarily responsible for importing British ideas into the United States. For example, he single-handedly popularized the British concept of the Enterprise Zone in the United States, and helped make it a viable political program.

In the United States, as in other countries, the most difficult federal programs to privatize are the entitlements programs (Social Security,

Medicare, Medicaid, and Aid to Families with Dependent Children.) Peter Ferrara's pathbreaking study of Social Security and follow-up studies by the Cato Institute have been extremely important in exposing the fact that the federal government's chain-letter approach to retirement pensions cannot survive and that there are practical, private alternatives. The NCPA's proposal to privatize Medicare (developed by Peter Ferrara, Gerald Musgrave, Richard Rahn and myself) already has generated considerable national political support, and legislation along these lines has been introduced into Congress.

Here, too, we have benefited from developments in Britain. In 1980 the American Enterprise Institute published a study by me on British Social Security. The study described a system under which British employers can contract their employees out of the second tier of the government's Social Security program by providing substitute private pensions that offer equal benefits. The British success with the program (over half of all British workers have been contracted out) adds considerable force to the argument for privatization of Social Security in the United States. Surprisingly, although my study was written for an American audience, it may have had greater political impact in Britain. I am told that it was a major factor in the Thatcher Administration's recent decision to completely privatize second tier pensions.

Washington does not lead; it follows. Rather than being the source of new ideas, Washington more often than not simply responds and reacts to them. It is for this reason, that the role of the think tank is so important. The Ed Feulners of this world are not answerable to voters. They do not have to worry about re-election campaigns. As a result, the major think tanks in the country can afford to propose ideas that are not immediately politically popular today—but which may succeed tomorrow. Ultimately, the think tanks, and the scholars and thinkers on which they rely, are the source of political change in this country.

It is therefore a heartening and welcome development to see major think tanks giving higher and higher priority to the concept of privatization. The Heritage Foundation has adopted privatization of federal programs as one of its major policy initiatives. The Reason Foundation remains in the forefront in pushing privatization at the local level. The National Center for Policy Analysis has started a three-year program to propose ways to privatize the entitlements programs and the federal welfare bureaucracy. The Competitive Enterprise Institute, under the leadership of Fred Smith, has played a central role in helping to forge coalitions in Washington to achieve practical political success. Of the many other institutes that are active in the privatization movement, the Cato Institute certainly deserves honorable mention. In addition there is the Political Economy Research Center, the Pacific Institute, the Manhattan Institute, Citizens for a Sound Economy, and many others.

We live in an era in which ideas are causing change. This volume represents a major step in the direction of explaining why and how it is happening.

John Goodman
Dallas, Texas
1985

Acknowledgements

This conference was designed to explore what is currently known about the theory and practice of privatization. Special thanks are due to Mr. and Mrs. Lovett Peters, without whose encouragement and support the conference would not have been held. We would also like to acknowledge a special debt to Richard Larry (Carthage Foundation) for his personal encouragement and to the Carthage Foundation for making the publication of this book possible.

Becci Breining and Carolyn Johnson were personally responsible for the organization of the conference (the skill and efficiency of their efforts was unanimously acknowledged) and along with Sue Mundell spent countless hours converting oral transcripts into a readable manuscript. We also would like to thank Bridgett Wagner (Heritage Foundation) and Willa Johnson (Willa Johnson & Associates) for their assistance in helping with the conference arrangements.

1

How Public Policy Institutes Can Cause Change

Ed Feulner

As the 98th Congress draws to a close, I am reminded of a statement Will Rogers made, which I can't help sharing. Mr. Rogers said, "I don't makes jokes—I just watch government and report the facts."

Ten years ago when the Heritage Foundation was started—conservatives were seen as wedded to "stale old ideas" from the past. We were opposed to change, our critics charged. We were told that we lacked a sophisticated understanding of the country's complex problems. In fact, we were often compared to the tailor who was lucky enough to have an audience with His Holiness the Pope and who, when asked afterward, "What's he like?" replied, "He's a 42 regular."

Conservatives were considered irrelevant by the opinion makers in the media, and the power brokers in the Congress ignored us. Now, many of those same Senators and Congressmen have entered involuntary retirement. Now, the Brookings Institute—the Liberals' favorite think tank—objects to being called "Liberal." I don't blame them.

Conservatives are supplying all of the new ideas—creative ideas—fresh in their approach to contemporary U.S. problems—but consistent with the basic, traditional values that have united us all these years.

We've certainly come a long way since Ronald Reagan first ran for Governor—thanks in large part to individuals all over the country like John Goodman and Stuart Butler, and thanks to institutions like National Center for Policy Analysis and the Heritage Foundation which we have helped build through our participation and financial support. But what does it take for public policy institutes such as the NCPA or my own Heritage Foundation to cause change in the political arena?

The Three I's: Ideas, Individuals and Institutions

Ideas. Many of you probably saw the *New York Times* Sunday Magazine article earlier this summer titled, "How New Ideas Shape Presidential Politics." In it, Walter Mondale's Issues Director is quoted as saying that "Ronald Reagan won last time on the strength of ideas."

Senator Moynihan, the eloquent Democrat from New York, confessed that the Republicans simply left the Democrats behind. The Republicans "Became the party of ideas and the Democrats were left, in Lord Macaulay's phrase, 'The stupid party.' There were ideas over there," said Moynihan, "So who ends up running the country? Politicians who know how to use ideas, that's who. The end product of government is laws—and laws emerge from ideas."

Individuals. Who produces ideas? Individuals. They also explain the ideas and expand them, but the third part of the equation is, if not the most important, the one I want to emphasize—the institutions.

Institutions. An individual needs an institutional base for support. An institution helps to popularize and propagandize the ideas. An institutional base provides more than just a paycheck to the individual. An institution has outreach capabilities to promote an idea on a continuing basis.

An institution should be large enough to have an "aura of authority," brash enough to come up with new ideas and not to be wed to the status quo. It should be principled enough to take on the establishment (like the steel industry on quotas) yet respectable enough to be considered seriously in the policy process. How does one move into the policy process? By shortening the path between the academic work done in the ivory towers and the practice of day-to-day governing.

Many have argued that the reason it has taken Professor Hayek's ideas so long to filter down to the general public and into the policy process is because he did not have an institutional base which would popularize and propagandize his ideas and provide a sense of continuity.

We have found that just producing ideas is not enough; they must be marketed. By the right people to the right people— largely the policymaking elite—in order to have an impact.

Who do we try to influence? Congress, the Administration and the national news media.

How do we influence these groups? Through the grassroots, the think tanks, the trade groups and the opinion leaders. We have learned that no matter how many studies you write or how beautifully they are printed, the effort is wasted if it has no impact on those who decide and implement policy.

Let me walk you through an example of how Heritage caused a change in the political arena.

We had an idea that the United Nations, like Pat Moynihan would say, is a "dangerous place." It has a budget of $4 billion—one-fourth of which the U.S.pays. It has 50,000 employees. One hundred fifty-eight nations represented, many with populations not much larger than this gathering. And what do we have to show for it? Resolutions denouncing Israel and South Africa, capitalism and the U.S.

So, in 1982 we formed our U.N. assessment project to see just what all this money went for. We now have two analysts, one research assistant and two distinguished senior fellows—Owen Harries, former Australian Ambassador to UNESCO and Charles Lichenstein, former alternate representative to the U.N. for political affairs.

Because of the number of complaints about UNESCO in our initial meetings with U.N. experts, UNESCO was a high priority project. We found UNESCO to be a wasteful, bloated bureaucracy; spending more on administration than on education, science or culture; biased against the U.S., the West and free enterprise; ruled by a third world majority dominated by the Soviet Union and radical socialist states.

We turned out six Backgrounders from October, 1982 to December, 1983 documenting our observations, with examples, numbers, names, UNESCO official resolutions and excerpts from their publications. Widespread press attention with luncheons, seminars, and workshops were organized to complement our work. We involved the key participants of the policymaking process; members of Congress, their staffs, Administration officials, press and representatives of organizations interested in the U.N.

Then, lo and behold, the mounting data began to change public opinion. This allowed for a whole new series of policy options to be considered. (In fact, the typically liberal press didn't rush to UNESCO's defense because of UNESCO's earlier attempts to impose a system of international quasi-censorship. Thus the press was neutralized.)

The U.S. has said that it will pull out of UNESCO at the end of this year. In the meantime the UNESCO operations have been audited by our own government to find out just what they have been spending all that money on. And certainly not to our surprise, the Government Accounting Office found that UNESCO is grossly mismanaged. It has enormous power vested in one man. Its governing bodies do not govern. There were no effective evaluating and coordinating systems. The programs had no clearly defined objectives and no target dates for completion. Hiring practices circumvented the organization's own regulations and undermined the professional integrity of the staff. There was little accountability for the money disbursed. There was an increasing concentration of staff at headquarters in Paris. Payments were being made in contravention of the organization's rules, and the recommendations of external auditors were repeatedly ignored.

The central role of The Heritage Foundation in all of this is well understood by UNESCO officials. They refused cooperation, refused to give us information, and even our publications requests were delayed. The Heritage Foundation was openly denounced by U.N. officials in discussion with diplomats at the U.N. I must admit that this is one of my very favorite examples of how the three "I's" have come together.

I have put together a short list of recommendations for what I would call marketing the product. These are some practical, nuts-and-bolts type suggestions that I'd like to share with you tonight. Work with the media, not against it. It does you no good to gratuitously slam them. Last summer, for instance, Richard Threlkeld did a five-minute special report about privatization on the ABC Nightly News. His treatment of the subject was overwhelmingly favorable, due in no small part to the fact that Steve Hanke, who was a Heritage Senior Fellow then and is now a Manhattan Institute Senior Fellow, was his primary source. The core idea behind this undertaking is the often unappreciated fact that articles and newscasts can vary immensely according to what sources were contacted. The first thing writers and producers need for a story is sources.

The second principle that we agreed on when the Heritage Foundation was established is what I call the "briefcase test." This principle is that studies should be as brief as possible. Arguments should be concise and clearly presented. Because of the vast number of issues addressed in Congress, there is a desperate need for concise studies which cut through the rhetoric and lay out the arguments succintly, to help members of Congress make informed choices on the issues before them. For this reason, we try to limit our *Backgrounders* to 10 pages—a document which stands a much greater chance of being put into the briefcase and read *before* the debate than a book which generally ends up on a bookshelf. We even have come up with an "urgent" format, the *Executive Memorandum*. This series outlines an argument in its briefest form—one sheet, front and back. *Executive Memorandum* is written, printed and hand-delivered to the relevant Washington offices in 24 hours, which often is all of the time left before a crucial decision is made.

Make contacts with speechwriting staff—on the local level and the national level. We are in touch with the Vice President's and the President's speechwriters. Once you get these ideas into speeches it is easier for those operating at the lower levels in the various departments to move an idea along.

A very good example of this was Enterprise Zones. It was part of the 1980 platform, the President has spoken of it in numerous speeches, and the proposal moved quite well through the Administration. Unfortunately, it has not done as well in the Congress. But, when the President begins to talk about a particular subject in his speeches, he moves an idea into the public debate. He helps to form the public opinion and in a sense he frames the debate.

This brings me to another point: Enlist support from a variety of sources. Even though this bill (Enterprise Zones) is still in Congress—it has passed the Senate and has more than 240 co-sponsors in the House and is supported by a majority on the House Ways and Means. However, we did not sit around and wait for Congress. Groups like the American Legislative Exchange Council and the Sabre Foundation have helped move the debates into the states. This has been a very effective maneuver: 23 states have now passed Enterprise Zone legislation. And Pennsylvania has Enterprise Zone administration policies in effect.

When possible, find out who is going to be affected by a certain policy and win their support *first* instead of coming out with a proposal and leaving these groups to react.

Take for example, privatization of public housing.

- The idea worked its way through the neighborhood-based organizations.

- We sent editorials out to the media.

- We picked up the support of Congressman Kemp, who has helped to push the idea and keep it out front.

- The proposal was included in the Republican Platform.

- Now the U.S. Department of Housing and Urban Development is working on a demonstration project.

Try to build "near beneficiary" groups. These are groups which don't quite qualify for a particular benefit, but would like to. These "near beneficiaries" help to build very effective lobbying efforts to expand a particular program.

For example, we have seen a big push for an expansion of IRAs to include nonworking spouses, and it has been very effective. Another example is the Enterprise Zone proposal: Once areas outside the zones realize how well the zones are doing with less taxation and less government intervention, they will press to have the zone expanded, or ask for the creation of a new zone for themselves.

Disseminate your ideas. We have had a number of successes in getting our ideas out through our journal *Policy Review*. By sending out press releases on certain articles, excerpting others, and encouraging op-eds, we have widened the market of these ideas and individuals. For example: George Gilder's "Triumph of the American Mind" was excerpted in the *Washington Times* (it took up an entire page), and was the subject of an important editorial on the semiconductor industry in the *Detroit News*, a column by nationally syndicated financial writer Robert Metz, and an editorial by the Voice of America. As a result of the article, Gilder was asked to appear on the MacNeil/Lehrer television program and twice on the Financial News Network.

Senator William Armstrong's "Therapy for the Budget" was the subject of a front-page news story and was excerpted in the *Washington Post's* editorial page "For the Record" section.

Adam Meyerson's article, "Elliott Abrams for Human Rights," was distributed by Congressman Jack Kemp to all Republican Congressmen through the House Republican Conference's News Summary. And, at a recent party in Managua, Mr. Abrams met the director of the North America desk for the Sandinista party. "Mr. Abrams," said the Sandinista, "I am so happy to meet you. I was just reading about you in *Policy Review*." So, we are widely read.

Certainly intellectual ideas can spread very quickly, yet their triumph at a particular time and place depends upon a variety of circumstances and accidents. For this reason, it is necessary to address a number of issues at the same time to be prepared to exploit circumstances which become ripe for influencing policy.

Always remember: Mainstream America and mainstream policymakers are receptive to conservative ideas and policies when properly exposed to them.

Right now we are at a crossroads in Washington.

What we have seen is that the right institutional support and institutional base can change the focus of debate on major political issues.

We have to have a legacy of our own institutions to outlast Ronald Reagan.

While we are riding the crest of the political wave, we should be building institutions for the next century. We should be using this time to establish conservative organizations.

Right now at Heritage we have a project which is encouraging a group we call the "Third Generation"—most of these people are under 30. We have held 18 meetings with speakers that include: Former New York Congressman John LeBoutillier; Grover Norquist, chief speechwriter and economist with the U.S. Chamber; and Frank Lavin, Deputy Director of the Office of Public Liaison in the White House. We average close to 100 attendees at each meeting.

As we have seen in the recent polls, Ronald Reagan's strongest support comes from the "Third Generation." The time to establish policies and organizations which include these people and which enable them to govern better is now.

You know we've come a long way when we start talking about a generation of conservatives. I think it's no accident that the younger people are more conservative in their political leanings. Conservatives *are* supplying the new ideas, and we've been able to popularize those ideas and move them into the political debate. And it's no accident that the younger people are excited about these new ideas.

Obviously, we now need to work to establish organizations like the National Center for Policy Analysis all over the country. And we need to continue holding conferences such as this where we can learn from our friends like Eamonn Butler and Madsen Pirie at the Adam Smith Institute. (Who by the way, have had more than their share of success stories.)

I think that if we move ahead keeping in mind the three "I's" that I mentioned earlier: Ideas, Individuals and Institutions, we will leave a legacy for this Third Generation which can carry the conservative movement into the next century.

2

Privatization Techniques and Results in Great Britain

Madsen Pirie

One of the great testaments to the great progress of the Thatcher Administration is that the word "privatization" (and indeed the idea of it) never appeared in the election manifesto of the Conservative Party in 1979. That election manifesto was a fairly traditional set of policies: To make government more cost effective, to cut the overall cost of government, to extend more choices to the people, and so on. But, the word privatization didn't appear.

Five years later in 1984, when British Leyland, the luxury car company that makes Jaguar was privatized, people were fighting in the streets to buy shares of stock. Television news coverage pictured gentlemen wearing bowler hats, bashing each other with brief cases and umbrellas, trying to get their share applications submitted in time. When the public starts fisticuffs, when there is brawling in the streets, when the city is brought to a halt by traffic jams, when thousands of people converge on a bank to buy shares of stock in a public company, obviously we have made some progress.

I am going to present a synopsis of the British privatization solution that was proposed or seriously considered and then rejected in favor of a non-traditional solution that worked. We have no shortage in Britain of people who say things like "We've got to get rid of the coal mines," or "We must denationalize the ports," or "The health service can't go on the way it is." We have no shortage of people like that and I imagine you are similarly well endowed in the United States with people who say "We've got to get rid of food stamps." Unfortunately, in the real world it doesn't work like that. You can't just go out and get rid of food stamps or denationalize industries. What we *are* short of in Britain is people telling us how to do it. And therefore, it is quite instructive to look at a series of cases in which the traditional proposal was set against the one that was actually successful.

Local Government Services

I will start with local government services, largely because we have made as much progress there as anywhere else and because it is an area which is often neglected. People from other countries often say that the scope of state ownership of industry and services is very small in their country. And it probably is small at the national level. Yet, it is at the local level of government in America and almost every advanced country in Europe that there is a very large degree of government ownership. Therefore, much progress can be made at this level in reducing public ownership.

What can be done about local government services? The traditional conservative answer has been to provide the services publicly and charge people fees for using them. Instead of providing services free at the point of consumption, such as free access museums, free street sweeping, free garbage collection, people are charged user fees. The theory is when you charge fees you impose economic disciplines. After all, if people are forced to pay for the service, they care about how much it costs. If they must pay users fees, they are going to regulate their demand. If the service is free, or at least free at the point of consumption, there is potentially no limit to the demand for the service. You could have garbage collectors calling three times a day, and indeed if it is free people may demand that level of service.

This traditional conservative solution was tried in Britain and it proved to be universally disastrous. It didn't work at all. It doesn't work because charging user fees has a political cost. Someone has to set these charges. When you fix the charges there is every pressure in the world to make them as low as possible and no pressure at all to keep them high. And so the pressure is on administrators and politicians to keep the charges as low as possible. Once those charges have been set, pressure is always to keep them low and to increase the size of the government subsidy. When those charges have to be renegotiated every year, politicians come under pressure from every conceivable interest. For example, when the time comes to set the charges for city bus services or refuse collection, city officials will be under considerable pressure from organized lobbies. Concerned citizens, senior citizens, the poor, the lame, the old—all will agree that their particular group should be exempted, that the charges must be kept low, and that an increase in fees would be absolutely wrong.

If the city officials try to hold out, if they try to stick to their principles and insist on charging fees which reflect true costs, they will be portrayed as somewhere between Scrooge and a Victorian Poor House manager, and they will be at serious risk in the next election. So it is a situation in which sound economic principles can be protected only by putting the best legislators at risk. There is every conceivable pressure on them to abandon their principles.

The alternative, which was adopted by the Thatcher Administration, was the contracting out of government services at the local level. That means having the service done by private business under contract to city government. The finance of the service is kept in the public sector, but the actual provision of the service is done by the private sector. Because there is competitive bidding, the private company providing the service faces constant pressure to keep costs down and quality high. This policy has saved local governments far more money than was ever saved by attempting to raise user fees. The policy also has proved to have few political costs, and it usually generates many political benefits.

The first local government in Britain to contract out one of its services was Southend Sea, which contracted out street cleaning and refuse disposal in 1980. Within six months, about half-a-dozen more cities contracted out services and another half-dozen followed six months later. Today, on the average one more city service somewhere is being privatized everyday. Everything ranging from architectural services to legal services, to pest control to grass cutting, to cleaning the public lavoratories, is now a candidate for privatization. And the amount of privatization has gone up spectacularly.

The labor unions last year earmarked 1.5 million pounds to campaign against privatization. But this is a drop in the bucket compared with the potential savings from privatization. We save 1.5 million pounds on a good contract in an average city. I might add that we also have gotten results without actually going to private contractors, but merely threatening to do so. In one case city workers who learned that their jobs were going to be put out for contract hastily huddled together and put in a bid and did exactly the same work at one-third less manpower. The savings were over one million pounds. When people come to us at the Adam Smith Institute from local government and ask how they can save money for their local governments, we always tell them simply to go back to council chambers and stand up and say the word "privatization." That alone will save them 20 percent. And if they go through with it, it will save them another 20 percent.

Public Housing

In Britain we have had housing problems in both the public and private sectors. The problem in public housing is that when Margaret Thatcher assumed office the government owned about 35 percent of all British housing units and more than one person in three lived in a publicly owned house at a highly subsidized rent. The rent was subsidized out of local property taxes paid by people who owned private houses. The problem with the private sector houses was rent control. It is universally enforced in Britain and it has kept rents below-market level. So with people living in public houses with below-market rents as well as people living in private houses with below market rents, you can appreciate why we had a housing shortage. It simply was not worth it to build new housing. People preferred to put their name on a waiting list for public housing and wait, because when they got it, it was so cheap and they could pass it on to their sons, their son's son and so on to the tenth generation. The situation was amazing. I still find it difficult to believe we actually did that, but we did.

The traditional policy of the Conservative Party in Britain for more than 20 years was to make public houses pay for themselves. Instead of giving subsidized rents, they proposed to raise the rents to economical levels. The Tories said this in every election and in every election they were beaten on the issue. And for a very good reason. The 35 percent of people living in those houses looked at the promises of the two candidates; one was saying we are going to give you cheap rent and the other was saying we are going to give you high rent. The tenants of these houses (called "council" houses) always chose the cheap rent, and they always voted that way. The Labour Party could regularly count on getting 90 to 95 percent of the votes from tenants of the public houses.

The Thatcher Administration tried a new tact. Instead of trying to make rents cover the cost of public housing, they decided to get rid of the houses by selling them to the tenants. The government recognized that a typical person living in a rented house probably would like to own it if they could afford to buy it, so the government offered them the right to buy.

In order to encourage sales, people were given the right to buy the houses at up to 50 percent off the market value depending on how long they had lived there. The Thatcher government realized it was worthwhile to do this because once people owned their own house there was no longer the problem of subsidized rent. So it is worth giving them half the value of the house in order to dispose of what otherwise was an annual loss to the government. Not surprisingly this proved to be successful. The tenants liked it because they could hold the house for a couple of years and then resell it for a profit. They could buy it for 20,000 pounds, wait two years and then sell it for 40,000 pounds.

What happened during the last election is that the Labour Party stood over on one side and said, "We will give you cheap rent," and the Tories stood on the other side and said, "We will give you free houses." The voters said, "We want the houses!" The Labour Party said they were going to take the houses back once they regained power. They now have officially and formally abandoned that position, for they realize there is a huge constituency out there who simply won't have anything to do with them if they threaten to take the houses away.

Of six million public housing units, about 250,000 have now been sold (about 15 percent) and sales are accelerating because the earlier sales occurred during a depression. We have the beginnings of an economic recovery in Britain and sales are up because people feel more confident in the future and in their ability to make mortgage payments. The government has increased the discount to 60 percent and introduced a new proposal for the people who cannot afford to buy them even at 60 percent off—a "part purchase," whereby people can buy part of their house. The idea is to get the houses out of the public sector at all cost, whatever it takes.

As far as Britain's private housing is concerned, the traditional policy always has been to abolish rent controls, and the Conservatives have gone to great lengths to do so. But they have tried repeatedly and failed. The reason they have failed is because there is a public outcry among the tenants and their lobbying organizations. And the weaker, less ideologically confident members of the Conservative Party wilt under this kind of fire and can't command a majority of the Legislature. So the attempts to abolish rent control have failed.

The Thatcher government introduced a new policy under which everyone who is in a rent control house can continue to enjoy rent controls, but any new property coming onto the market can be let without rent control. The idea is quite specifically to set in motion a chain of events that will lead to the end of rent control. People who live in rent control houses are not threatened. When the new policy was enacted there were no marches in the streets; there were no demonstrations. The act was put through Parliament on a quiet Wednesday afternoon without anyone noticing.

Not one new property in the whole of Britain has come onto the market under rent control since this policy was adopted. Every single new property which comes onto the market comes under leases negotiated in the free market. As people in rent control houses die, as they move away, or as their landlords buy them out, the property moves into the free market. So the portion of property under rent control is declining steadily and will continue to decline until there is none left. Now *that*, you see, is a different type of approach. Everyone who has enjoyed the privilege has been guaranteed that privilege will continue. The existing generation is being bought out so the change can be effective for the next generation.

Health Care

The National Health Service costs an enormous amount of money. The quality of service is getting worse, there is a lot of unnecessary and wasteful spending, and much of the benefits go to those who don't need subsidies from government. The traditional Conservative policy in Britain has been to try and weed out and take away benefits from those who don't need them and, achieve administrative savings by cutting out waste. There always has been a public outcry, with television news programs showing how the new policies are having devastating effects on the poor.

The same thing has happened to President Reagan in this country. He has been cast as someone who is attempting to save money by taking away the benefits from the poor and giving tax advantages to the rich, even though the policy changes were enacted in order to make the system more rational and cost effective. What begins as an attempt to cut out the most extreme absurdities of waste ends up being portrayed on CBS News that night as an attempt to put widows and disabled people out onto the streets in the snow. Of course the politicians quickly respond by deploring the new policies.

The same thing happened in Britain. The attempt to cut or to cut out waste always failed. So the Thatcher government has embarked on a new strategy: to deliberately foster private alternatives that will encourage people to leave the state sector *by choice*. The British have been telling themselves for years that we have the finest health service in the world, which cares for people from cradle to grave or, as they say these days, from pre-natal to county crematorial. Yet people are now leaving it in droves. The number of people with private insurance in Britain has gone through the roof. And it has spread into trade union negotiations to the extent that private insurance is now part of collective bargaining. Today there are about 600,000 union members covered by private health insurance.

About 4.2 million people in Britain pay for state services through their taxes. If they want to use private insurance as well, they have to pay twice. They end up paying once for the state service they don't use, and once for the private service they do use. Not surprisingly, this means that the choice thus far has existed only for the rich—those who could afford to pay twice. The Thatcher government introduced a principle of giving tax benefits to people who opted out. If you take private insurance you are saving the state money in the National Health Service, so it gives you back a little bit of that money you saved them. That little bit is your incentive, which makes it that much cheaper for you to take the private alternative. This is only one tiny hole in the dam, but it's getting bigger. Once the principle is established, arguing about the price is the only thing that remains.

George Bernard Shaw, in conversation with a lady at dinner, asked if she would accompany him to bed for a million pounds. She said yes. He then asked if she would accept only five pounds. Insulted, she said, "What do you think I am?!" To which he replied, "We've already established what you are, we are now arguing about the price." A similar principle applies to opting out and encouraging exit. Once the principle has been conceded, we are now talking about the price.

Education

The traditional conservative proposal has been the voucher system. Vouchers give parents choice. It is a very good idea, and if we all woke up tomorrow morning and found vouchers in progress it would be a marvelous world. Unfortunately, it has been proposed many times and never succeeded in getting off the ground. The voucher idea has been around for more than 60 years, and there have been numerous attempts to get a trial scheme put into effect. Unfortunately, the vouchers alienate parents because they don't understand what sounds to them like some crazy idea, and because they fear they are going to lose the free place their children have at their local school. Teachers, of course, are determined to oppose vouchers, for it will mean losing control. The local authorities who administer the schools also see in vouchers a loss of power. So every single group you can think of in the education process is opposed.

So vouchers are an excellent idea, but politically they are just not feasible. The solution is one which involves giving the parents control over the schools—that is, having schools run by boards of parents. If you have a child at the school, you get a vote. In addition, parents on the school board are given the power to hire and fire the principal and other members of the faculty. Combine with that the finance of schools on a capitation basis, based on the number of children in the school. Now if you add the right to move your child to the school of your choice, you begin to see emerging a radically different educational system.

Under the new system if parents don't like a particular school, they can move their child elsewhere. As the child moves elsewhere, the school's capitation goes down by one. If they have one less child, they get a little bit less money. The new school to whom the child is sent sees its roll go up by one; and it receives a little bit more money. With parent control of the schools, there is the possibility that the schools will begin to vary. Some may achieve academic excellence, and stress traditional pursuits. Others may adopt the latest sociological theory and allow the children to pour glue into each others ears in the name of encouraging uninhibited creativity. The parents will, I imagine, desert these schools in droves. The schools, in other words, will have to compete for customers in much the same way that business firms compete in the marketplace.

The obvious questions can be asked: "How does this differ from the vouchers?" The answer is: "Not at all." This is the solution I think we're going to see tried in Britain.

Regulatory Agencies

In the United States you have regulatory agencies. We in Britain have QUANGOS. A QUANGO is an acronymn for quasi-autonomous, non-governmental organization. They are bodies appointed by government, but not directly answerable to Parliament. They are a kind of para-bureaucracy. We discovered there were 3,068 of these bodies, staffed by tens of thousands of bureaucrats. The traditional conservative policy has been: "When we take over, we're going to put the right people in." And when the right people were put in, they became the wrong people very rapidly. You put the "right" people in, and lo and behold they somehow find that the arguments they previously had for getting rid of these agencies and doing away with their work are no longer persuasive.

The alternative of the Thatcher government is to replace QUANGOS with private alternatives. Twenty percent of these bodies have been replaced with private, voluntary substitutes. For example, there originally were three QUANGOS related to birds: the Advisory Committee on Bird Sanctuaries in the Royal Parks, the Advisory Committee on the Protection of Birds in England, and the Advisory Committee on the Protection of Birds in Scotland. The government was advised that the Royal Society for the Protection of Birds (RSPB) was an independent body funded by subscriptions from its members, and was, in fact, better than all of the other three put together. The RSPB gave consistently better advice, and therefore was a better body to deal with. The government transferred to the RSPB the bird sanctuaries that were previously administered by the three QUANGOS.

Of the 3,068 QUANGOS in existence when Margaret Thatcher took office, a little more than 600 have been privatized or abolished. That is a 20 percent reduction, quite good for one term in office. But, of course, much more remains to be done.

Nationalized Industries

In Britain there are many regulations which limit industrial development. What does a person opening a business have to go through? If you attempt to open a business in Britain, you direct your request to the Department of Industry. You are supplied with all the regulations that have to be met: health and safety, building standards, and rules like: "The fire extinguisher shall be affixed to the wall." It is the same with the Occupational Safety and Health Administration in the U.S.

The traditional policy has been to attempt to repeal these regulations, and it is very tough going. Regulatory agencies have a mind of their own. You have to fight for a long, long time, to battle for two or three years to get one minor change, such as modifying the rule about how lavoratory seats must be made. After winning the battle, you are allowed some variety of choice as to whether to use plastic or wood. But it is very debilitating to undertake this kind of fight. You get bogged down in detail and end up thinking it is a great victory if three years later you've got some minor paragraph inserted into the Federal Registry.

The solution we tried in Britain is to establish experimental areas of deregulation. The idea is to prove in selected areas that if you do away with all the regulation it doesn't result in Mongol hoards sweeping in from the East. Life goes on. Industry is more successful. We're optimistic that once we have proven on a small scale that deregulation can lead to improvements, everyone will want to get in on the act.

What do you do with these state-owned industries? If the company is making a profit, traditional Tory policy has been to leave it alone on the grounds that we can use the money. The conservative policy has been if it is making a loss, we can't get rid of it. A minority of Conservatives did argue that profitable firms should be sold. They said, "If it is making a profit today, it will surely make a loss tomorrow. Let's get rid of it while it is still profitable." But, they wanted to sell to a private buyer.

What the Thatcher government did instead was to sell to the public. The policy was to issue stock and invite the public to buy. And so the British public is buying large shares in British Telecom, British Leyland, and on and on. There are four pages packed with titles of companies of various sizes that have been sold to the public. What this means is that the public now has a vested interest in keeping these companies in private hands, and any Labour government that wants to take them back again under state ownership will find the general public a very effective opposition lobby.

There were many state industries that were making a loss. These could not be sold in the same way. The traditional Conservative policy has been to close them down. This meets with a lot of opposition in the workforce. It meets with strikes, sit-ins, marches in the streets, and television documentaries on the potential harm. It is an unrewarding approach. What the Thatcher government did instead was to promote a worker buy-out, which has been an extraordinary success story. For example, the National Freight Corporation, the government's trucking company, was making horrendous losses. The government sold it to the employees, with much of the money coming from the employer's pension funds. It has been a spectacular success every year since then. Its annual reports show profits, with the employee-held shares increasing enormously in value. The workers used to spend their time fighting over who was allowed to do which job, disputes which characterize state industries in Britain. They are now so busy making money hand-over-fist and satisfying consumers that they have no time for these little disputes. It is a formula that is being applied more and more to a variety of industries.

Subsidies

Subsidized activities, such as school meals in Britain, are state provided at highly subsidized rates. Meals that cost about 60 pounds are provided by the state to children for 20 pounds, with the taxpayer picking up the difference. If you try to justify the state subsidy you get nowhere at all. If you try to withdraw the subsidy you get howls of hysterical protest. The new Thatcher policy has been to contract on the basis of least subsidy. You announce the service that needs to be provided, school meals for children, for example, and discover who can do it for the least subsidy. Firms bid against each other to see who can do it for the lowest price, requiring the least amount of taxpayer revenues.

The policy has been very successful. The cost of school meals has gone down and the quality has gone up. When the meals were provided by state workers, the children used to get a kind of brown goo on a plate. They now serve better meals and the children have more choices. It has been a total success. The only people objecting are the ladies who used to do it, and most of those have been hired by the private companies.

Utilities

In Britain, the big utilities are state-owned monopolies. These include gas, electricity, and the telephone service. The traditional Conservative approach has been to try to divide them up by geographic areas. Telephone service, they said, is a natural monopoly: You can't have two sets of telephone wires going into the same house. Gas also is a natural monopoly. You can't have two gas pipes going into the same house. So the Conservative proposal was to divide the country up into areas, so that the performance in one area could be compared with the performance in another. Under this approach differences in performance would lead to embarrassing questions: Why are you in West Yorkshire charging 4.5 pence per therm when down in the East they're managing to do it for 3.3 pence per therm? Obviously, you're operating inefficiently.

The idea never got anywhere. The gas boards and the electric boards proved themselves quite capable of resisting it. They said they need to operate on a national scale in order to take full advantage of economies of scale. It was a very effective argument.

The Thatcher government chose a different approach. It repealed the monopoly status of the utilities. The government simply has said that anyone who wants to supply gas can do so. Anyone who wants to supply electricity can do so. Anyone who wants to supply telephone equipment can do so. What is happening is in several areas is that the monopoly is being eroded by repealing the monopoly protections, rather than attempting to break the monopoly up. This is particularly true in the case of telephones. I doubt that British Telecom now supplies a majority of the telephones sold in the United Kingdom, and that is within two years of losing its monopoly status. Four years ago, every telephone in Britain was a black thing with a dial in the middle—just like it was in the 1930s. In four years the market has changed enormously. Britain is now almost as advanced as the U.S. in radio phones and other innovations, all as a result of the repeal of the monopoly.

Other Government Services

In Britain if you live in public housing (more than five million people still do) the state maintains your house. It comes and fixes pipes and windows and performs other maintenance duties. The water supply in Britain is nationalized; broken mains and faucets have to be repaired by the state. The traditional Conservative policy has been to try to make these services more efficient. They have set up Use Accounts so that consumers, meeting together, can exercise a voice and report that the service isn't really satisfactory. Unfortunately, they end up being captured by the industry that they are supposed to be against. We now have the total absurdity of the Use Accounts *endorsing* increases in postal charges on the grounds that it will give customers a better service!

The new policy, which has just been introduced, is to give people the right of private substitution in the event the state service fails. The new housing bill has this written into it. If you want to have your state-owned house repaired privately, you call in private contractors, have it fixed, and then bill the state. The same principle is going to be used in the water industry. If your local water main bursts, and they don't fix it, you bring in private plumbers, get the thing fixed and then bill the government. You have the right to have the repairs and maintenance done privately and have the government pay for it if it fails to fulfill its statutory obligation.

Conclusion

There are four major areas of the public sector which are candidates for privatization in Britain. 1. nationalized industries, 2. utilities (gas, electricity, telephones, etc.), 3. regulatory bodies, and 4. social services (health care, pensions, etc.). I have listed them in order of the difficulty of privatizing them.

The greatest progress has been made in the first category, through the sale of state industries. But substantial progress also has been made in each of the other areas. The Thatcher government has demonstrated that no areas of the public sector is immune to the wave of privatization which is sweeping Britain.

I have given you a number of case histories, covering each of the four public sector areas. In each case I have contrasted the traditional approach (which did not work) with the Thatcher government's approach (which did work). These case histories and many more are described in detail in my book *Dismantling the State: The Theory and Practice of Privatization.*

Some people look at Britain and suppose that privatization merely means selling off state assets. That is wrong. Privatization in Britain as practiced by the Thatcher Administration means having done privately that which was previously done publicly. It does not matter if it is a regulatory function, health, education, industries, or utilities. In Britain, privatization is an approach. It is not a message or a policy. It is a determination to approach the public sector as an enemy and to get rid of it piece by piece.

We already have won the intellectual battle in Britain. We also have identified our policies with the future. People generally believe that as a manufacturing economy changes to a service and high-tech economy, our policy of choice, variety, and opportunity is more appropriate to the future. The Left and the collectivists are reeling at the moment, trying to conserve a way of life that the general public sees as dying away. I would not want to be in their position.

3

How the Thatcher Revolution was Achieved

Eamonn Butler

I want to discuss the kind of strategies by which privatization was put into practice in Britain. This involves not just the ideas themselves, but the mechanisms and procedures that we have been using to get those ideas across, to get them taken seriously, and then to get them put into practice.

The first thing that I must stress about the Thatcher privatization revolution is that it was not something that was done by careful planning, certainly not on the part of the politicians! When Mrs.Thatcher took office, there was in the party platform a commitment to lowering public expenditures, but nothing at all about contracting out government services. And amazingly, contracting out local government services has been one of the government's strongest achievements, while its efforts to lower public expenditures has not been as successful.

When Thatcher took office in 1979, many conservatives thought that it would be very easy to reduce government expenditure by techniques such as cutting out waste. I'm sure that American politicians, too, like to cut out waste. Before the election British politicians made pious statements about how much waste there was in bureaucracy. Many other people thought that you could simply go in with a hatchet and cut down government programs right, left and center, and that you could enforce cash limits on the budgets of nationalized industries and thus bring them under control. Of course, none of this was achieved. The level of public expenditure in Britain today is not very much different from what it was in 1979.

According to traditional conservative thinking, politicians need only to be *determined* enough; they have to have the political "will" to go in and cut the public sector. Well, I've never actually seen political "will." And you can't expect politicians to volunteer to make themselves unpopular by reducing government programs that benefit a lot of people. The beneficiaries are not only the people who are receiving benefits from the program but also the people who are running the programs. Trying to get politicians to cut programs is rather like trying to get turkeys to discuss the merits of an early Thanksgiving!

Making Small Changes

Consequently, sweeping cuts have proved impossible. But there have been a large number of things that have happened on a small scale, what we call the micro-political scale, since small-scale changes have the potential to develop into much larger changes later on. Small starts were made with ground being broken in lots of different areas. It is very appropriate that this paper should be entitled "The Thatcher Experiment," because a great many of the things that have been quite successful started out simply as experiments.

Progress started to be made by tackling the easy targets first. We had a government in 1979 which was very committed and ideological but, very wisely, decided that it would not immediately take on many of the things that its supporters wanted it to take on. Many of its supporters in 1979 thought that the first thing we ought to do was to go in and break up the unions. This is because the unions were seen, and are still seen by many people in Britain, as being the greatest threat to any progress in the United Kingdom. The government appointed a very soft man to tackle the union problem. A little bit was done but not very much. Then the next year a little bit more was done. The next year a bit more still. And so at the end of four or five years, we now have a policy on trade unions which I think is almost as rigorous as those which the conservative hard-liners were suggesting that we should have adopted in 1979. But it happened gradually, without the unions themselves being able to organize very much effective opposition against it. The strategy was just one small change after another that no one felt particularly strongly about.

The government also approached the issue of the National Health Service very wisely. The attitude of the Minister of Health was "I did not come into office in order to preside over the dismantling of the National Health Service." The National Health Service concept of free medical care for everybody is such an entrenched idea in Britain that it would have been very unwise for the government to simply cut out benefits right away. So there was not an immediate attack on the Health Service as some conservatives had proposed. Instead, competition has been encouraged, private contractors are taking over ancillary services, and charges for NHS treatment have been raised gradually.

There were a number of very small things that had very significant effects in other fields. For example, one of the first actions of the government was to deregulate the bus services between cities. This has been a very interesting experience because the deregulation of buses between cities has led to an enormous improvement in services; it led to fare reductions of about 50 percent on most services, and it has resulted in the delightful but unexpected by-product of our state railroad company coming under serious competitive threat from all of these booming private sector bus companies. Who would have thought that buses would introduce videos and stewardess services, and make so much improvement in service that they would put very strong economic pressure on the railroads? (That, of course, is making it easier to deal with the powerful rail unions.)

The experience has been so good over the last three or four years that we are now going to do exactly the same thing on urban buses. Instead of being run by the local governments, in the future they are going to be broken up and run by private firms. The Adam Smith Institute played some part in that: A while ago we published a book on bus deregulation, looking at practical examples throughout the world, and that led to the government white paper on bus deregulation. The laws that will follow it probably will be enacted in November and December of 1984. So the Thatcher program has been rather opportunistic; it has been a gradualist program which developed as it went along. Instead of trying to enforce sweeping and rigid changes, it has taken advantage of the opportunities that small changes have produced.

Creating Freedom of Choice

A very important aspect of how the Thatcher experiment was achieved was to give people a taste of free choice. We can argue; we can write books; we can give seminars about the advantages of freedom and free enterprise. But what actually changes people's minds? It is being able to buy health care privately instead of having to wait six months for an operation in a National Health Service hospital. It is being able to travel by a bus, cheaply, with lots of competition, rather than being dependent upon one state-operated bus company. It is the taste of being able to own your own home rather than to have to rent it from the government, and the taste of being able to do things with that home under private ownership.

All of these things give people their first taste of the market economy. They begin to understand this new-found freedom and say to themselves, "Actually, it's not bad." And then you can build on that and do yet more to introduce further competition.

As part of our work designed to encourage people to think about the value of freedom, we discovered there were 252 kinds of government inspectors who had the power to come into your home or your office, take your papers away and photocopy them, and invade your personal liberty in other ways. We always thought that an Englishman's home was his castle. But no, there are 252 different ways of getting into that private castle. And so we published a list of these agencies, and we presented it like a restaurant guide—with little symbols beside each agency's name. There was an ax if they could break the door down, and there was a filing cabinet if they could take your papers away, and so on. That helped enormously. We were quite surprised to be called in by a government official who said, "The Prime Minister has put me in charge of cutting down these inspections." He had our book in front of him. And he opened it and said, "Now, where shall we start?"

The point of this example is that very often politicians want people to tell them what to do! They know the goal they want to reach, but they don't know how to get there.

The Role of Think Tanks

One other thing instrumental in helping the Thatcher achievements was positive backing from British think tanks. It had the good fortune of having many think tanks that were exploring these ideas, that knew something about the political process and how to influence it.

The support has not come from traditional sources. For example, the Confederation of British Industry, which is a federation of employers, came into open conflict with the government on the subjects of inflation and recession. They wanted inflationary budgets because their pockets were torn. They openly attacked the government saying, in effect, that more public spending was needed. They did not want to lose government contracts. They wanted Mrs.Thatcher to keep spending high. What happened was that they quickly became ineffective.

On the other hand, an organization that did support our efforts, the Institute of Directors, came in with very effective media presentations. Their work filled the void. They are now active privatizers, with good policy analysis teams who we work with very closely. They are very effective at presenting themselves. The government now is finding that under this remorseless pressure the range of options that politicians have to choose from becomes wider and wider from the right, when it used to be from the left.

Politicians like this. There is nothing worse if you are a politician than to have to stand and announce some new policy that no one has ever heard of before, even if it is 100 per cent sound economics. But if there are 30 or more think tanks putting out the same idea in advance, he can announce a new policy everyone has heard before in the media. The politician then can stand up and note that all of the experts agree to support this good idea, which has been in general circulation for some years.

So a very strong component in the Thatcher Administration, I think, has been taking new ideas from think tanks. This has been a particularly effective weapon in the Thatcher experiment.

Media Relations

The government itself has used a professional public relations team for the first time since the 1979 election. At first it was frowned upon, but it has proved to be very effective. And think tanks like ours also have been getting more experience at using media. You have to work with the media, not in opposition to it. I am very lucky because part of my time I am an editor of a magazine. I have to think like a journalist; and, therefore, I know what journalists are like. Like the rest of us, they are lazy, but they have a job to do, and have to supply their editors with good copy.

You have to see a problem from their point of view. If you have something to say, you have to package it in a way that allows a busy journalist to grasp the point quickly and not spend a lot of time rewriting your press release. Also, you would not get him to respond by bombarding him with information packets and huge reports and thinking that he is going to read them. And you won't do it by giving him something that is outdated or so unnewsworthy that there is no "peg" to hang it on. You are not going to get him to use your material if there is no clear story.

It is particularly important to have a battery of experts for the news media to contact. You might get a phone call from a journalist saying, "We are thinking of doing a story on rent control." You should be able to say, "Good. There are five people you can call and speak to on that. Here are their names and telephone numbers." That is very effective. If the media taps several experts in several organizations it looks as though there is an enormous wave of opinion out there. I realize that the situation in Britain is different from the United States because we have national TV, national radio, and national newspapers, all headquartered in London. If the Adam Smith Institute gets an idea into the *Daily Mail*, and the *Express*, we have got that story into about two-thirds of all British households. It is very easy for us to do that, but it is not done simply by bombarding them. It is done by working with them—by calling on the appropriate people and floating the story, and suggesting a way in which it might be done.

Effective use of the media can be accomplished in another way! Madsen Pirie writes many articles for one of our leading newspapers, the *Daily Mail*. What he used to do is sit down with the editor over lunch and say, "I have a list of 20 ideas that I think would make good feature articles. Which ones do you want?" He got the editor's input about the ideas he thought were the best. The editor decided to use them because after that they became his idea, rather than Madsen's. It is amazing what can be accomplished using this approach.

One of those lunches occurred just after the government announced it was considering a policy we had proposed. The policy was: Instead of spending public money to build highways, the government would have private firms finance the new roads and be repaid by the government on the basis of how much the roads are used. Well, at this lunch, the editor of *Daily Mail* finally got around to saying, "Before we do anything else, I want to apologize. Six months ago you came to me with your list of topics and one of them was private roads. I said, 'Oh, that's too zany. That will never happen. I was wrong.' " So good ideas *can* get through.

Small-Scale Experiments

As well as seeing things from the point of view of the journalist, I think you also see things from the point of view of politicians. Experiments are of value in this. It is very difficult to oppose an experiment. Few vested interest groups are going to oppose small experiments here and there to determine whether a theory works.

These experiments can be effective. We originally suggested the Enterprise Zone experiment, but in Britain the idea never caught hold because the civil service opposed it from the beginning, and the government ministers did not have the political base to resist the civil service pressure to water the idea down. So we said, "All right, let us have some more experiments—Freeport experiments—and have an actual fence of demarcation around it so we can charge different tax rates, we can have different employment legislation, and so on." This experiment was more successful; we now have six Freeports. They are only an experimental basis, but if each works we might do it elsewhere. It is very difficult for organizations to resist these kinds of small-scale experiments.

Building Coalitions

Isaac Newton scholars will recognize the phrase "minimum necessary change." This is what we're always aiming for. We look for the minimum change that we need in order to have an effect later on. We want something that is going to seem reasonable to the general public. And we want something that is going to be reasonably easy to do, which then can grow.

Take, for example, the tax deduction for people who buy private health insurance. At first it is introduced in a tiny way, so that few opponents will notice. Then the deduction is expanded and more and more people begin to buy private health insurance. The whole thing gradually builds up to the point where your little acorn has now become a big oak tree putting shade over the public sector services and causing them to wither away. I am sure that Americans will know the importance of building up forces in a coalition.

The public housing tenants who have purchased their own housing units are now an important lobby group. People who own the property that was once owned by the government do not want to see it taken away. Shareholders in newly privatized national industries are another example. The British government has gone to great lengths to be sure that when it sells shares they get into as many hands as possible.

Denationalization started when shares were sold in a few companies. But there were complaints that the professional business investors bought up all of the shares, while the ordinary man in the street did not actually buy very much. This meant that ownership in the denationalized company was concentrated in the hands of a small group, which lacked the political clout to protect the company against the possibility of re-nationalization at some future date. So in the case of British Telecom, our state telephone service, the sale was done through merchant banks, which spent millions on TV and print advertising appealing to the ordinary members of the public. And the ads all said, "It is your phone company. Why not buy a share in it?" In fact the ads said even more: "If you do buy a share in it, we will give you a discount on your phone bill." Now that is the sort of thing that the ordinary man in the street can understand. His reaction is, "Right. I'd like to buy one of these shares if I can get 20 percent off my phone bill."

Whether the ordinary American public thinks they are getting the full advantage of the various privatizations that are going on, I do not know. In Britain they do because they can see it. They can ride the buses, they can buy the shares, and they can see the benefits they are getting. Cultivating the involvement of the man in the street is very important.

Buying off the people who are affected by change is equally important. We have reduced the civil service in our country from around 700,000 to roughly 600,000. We have not done it just by firing them all. We have done it by very generous retirement plans and by paying severance benefits—in some cases, quite stupendous amounts of money. But it is worth spending the money to get them out of the public sector so they are no longer part of a vested interest lobby group.

Packaging Ideas

When introducing new policies you have to be intelligent in the way you present them. It is no good, for instance, to say, "Welfare benefits ought to be cut." Even if I thought welfare benefits ought to be cut, I would not say that. What I would say instead is we need welfare reform, that we need rational spending and that the money we save can be used either for reducing taxes or, even better, to improve the lot of the truly needy. It is all in how you present the idea. The same policy is just dressed up in a different way.

The things you promote ought to be based on some measure of the practical. Many areas in which we have had the greatest success are areas where we have pointed to the practical experience of other countries. An ounce of practice is always worth a pound of theory. This is why I am eager to build up the international links between all of the institutes on our side,because I think that in foreign countries you often can find practical experience to support what you have been proposing in theory.

Gradualism

In Britain we have a group called The Fabian Society, which was set up in 1884. Their slogan is, "The inevitability of gradualism." They reckoned that when you take on a little bit at a time you gradually wear down the stone. Well, we are doing exactly the same, but in the opposite direction. We are building up new coalitions, and the opposition does not like it.

You must not assume that the people you think are your enemies really are. There is talk about the American news media being very left-wing, and that is true. We have exactly the same problem, not necessarily in our newspapers but certainly in our radio and television media. We have a state-owned broadcasting company, after all. These people are paid by the state. They are not exactly going to queue up to be broad-minded about privatization. Yet, by presenting the ideas in the right way, by being reasonable and understanding of the problems of those who are going to be displaced when privatization happens, and by building elements in the new policies that take care of them and recognize their interests, we can achieve a great deal.

4

Privatization in the U.S.: Why It's Happening and How It Works

John C. Goodman

There is a way of thinking about the political process that has greatly influenced American free-market economists. It has probably influenced to a great extent every participant in this conference. For lack of a better term, I will call it "public choice theory." I feel that in order to really appreciate privatization and how it works, we have to modify our thinking a bit about this theory.

The conventional way of thinking about public choice theory in the United States involves accepting three propositions. The first is the idea that there is a winning platform. This is the position on all issues which is the best position in terms of winning elections. If there is one best position on all of the issues, the candidates will, out of necessity, tend to endorse this platform. If one candidate endorses this platform and his opponent does not, the candidate who fails to adopt the winning platform will lose the election. The implication of this proposition is that politicians have very little choice about what they do.

A second proposition that characterizes American public choice thinking is that in our political system arbitrarily redistributes incomes. By arbitrary redistribution of income I mean taking money out of the pockets of some and giving it to others, for no other reason than the fact that the receiving group has more votes or more political power than the groups whom they plunder. Most economists not only view the political world this way, but they almost take it for granted that everyone else views it this way, too.

In other words, if you are going to have a political system in which people have an unrestricted right to vote on economic issues, then they are going to vote in an unrestricted way on economic issues. And more likely than not, they will vote for policies that are in their self-interest. The bottom line will be that you will have all kinds of income transfers. Agricultural policies, for example, will transfer income out of the hands of consumers and into the hands of farmers. Tariffs, regulations, and other public policies similarly serve to make some people better off at the expense of others. Combined with the assumption of the winning platform, that is what this idea implies. There always will be one "best way" of redistributing income in the political sector which politicians will tend to endorse. The theory also assumes that there is always an infinitely elastic supply of politicians willing to endorse any platform to get elected. If one office-holder refuses to carry out the winning platform, there is always some other politician willing to replace him who will do so.

A third proposition of American public choice theory is the proposition that individual politicians "don't matter." In economics we have the theoretical notion of the Walrasian auctioneer. This is a mythical figure who somehow makes supply equal demand in all markets. In other words, he chooses the "right price" so that there is equilibrium in every market. In political theory we have a similar notion of equilibrium. We are in political equilibrium when we have the right position on all issues—in other words, when the winning platform is being enacted into law.

The difference between economic theory and political theory is that in political theory, the auctioneer is somebody real—he is a politician. He is the individual who chooses the winning platform and captures the election. I think we need to modify our thinking on these propositions in order to appreciate the phenomenon of privatization.

Let us begin with the notion of redistributing income. It is not clear to me that the American people have ever accepted the principle of arbitrary redistribution of income. In our book, *Economics of Public Policy*, Ed Dolan and I discussed a hypothetical bill to aid wealthy farmers. The bill proposes to impose a tax on consumers—a regressive tax which takes proportionately more from the poor than from the rich. The money goes into a fund called The Fund for Wealthy Farmers. This money is distributed to farmers in such a way that almost all of it goes to the rich farmers and only a little trickle goes to poor farmers. In the book we asked whether such a bill could ever make its way through Congress. Our answer was: no. It could never get through Congress, even though what I have just described is the practical consequence of American agricultural policy.

If you stop to think about it, you have never heard Walter Mondale say,

"When elected, I am going to take $30 billion out of the hands of consumers and give it to the farmers. The reason I am going to do this is that farmers have their act together and they can deliver more electoral votes. Four years from now, if you consumers can get your act together, and if you are a little better organized, maybe you will lose only $15 billion." We have never heard him say that, and I think that is not a trivial point. The reason we never hear this kind of rhetoric is that the voting public does not accept the principle of arbitrary redistribution of income. I am reminded of the McGovern demogrants—a proposal to give every American $1,000 and then raise the tax rates for high-income taxpayers. Remember how shocked people were at this proposal? People who would have gained by the proposal voted against George McGovern. There is no better evidence that the American public does not generally accept the principle of arbitrary redistribution of income.

The public goes along with programs which arbitrarily redistribute income because they are tricked or fooled into believing there is an underlying social purpose, such as the notion that the program will get us out of depression, or help our national defense, or achieve some other social goal. If I am correct, if that is what has been going on, then that means there is a lot of room on our side of the issue for our own tricking and fooling. Or, to put it differently, there are ways of recasting issues to bring about change.

Consider the idea of the "winning platform." I believe we have been too narrow in our thinking. We have failed to consider the possibilities for innovation in this area.

Figure I depicts the issue of British public housing rents. This is a one-dimensional graph representing a single issue. The issue is how high the rent will be. On the right is the highest possible rent and on the left is the lowest possible rent. The figure also depicts three groups in their functional roles and what their positions are. On the right are the taxpayers who want rents kept high so taxes will be kept low. On the left are rentpayers and the public housing bureaucracy, the people who want rents kept low. We also might put here the idealists—those people who in principle are opposed to private property.

Figure II depicts the same graph with a new issue added, the proposal to sell the houses to tenants at greatly reduced prices. To think of this new issue required innovative thinking on the part of the Thatcher Administration. So the second new issue is: to sell the houses or not to sell them. Now we have a four-quadrant diagram with four possible political positions, and the coalition on the left has been divided. The heavy dark spot shows what was previously the political equilibrium, the winning platform. The dark arrow shows how the winning platform changes through time.

The public housing bureaucracy is down in the lower left quadrant. It wants low rents and does not want the houses sold, because then public housing authorities will not have anything to administer. Rentpayers, on the other hand, are at the top left hand quadrant. They want low rent, but they also gain by the right to buy. The resulting split allows for political movement, for change through time. The houses are not sold all at once, but as more and more rentpayers buy, the number of individuals beginning to think like taxpayers swells. This changes the political equilibrium.

Figure I

PUBLIC HOUSING: ONE DIMENSIONAL ISSUE GRAPH

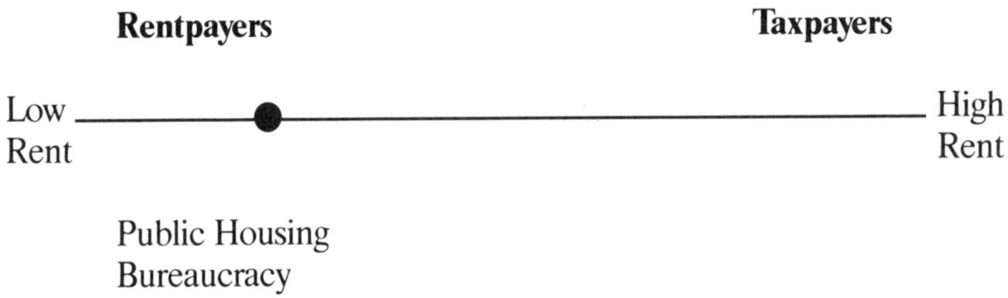

Figure II

PUBLIC HOUSING: TWO DIMENSIONAL ISSUE GRAPH

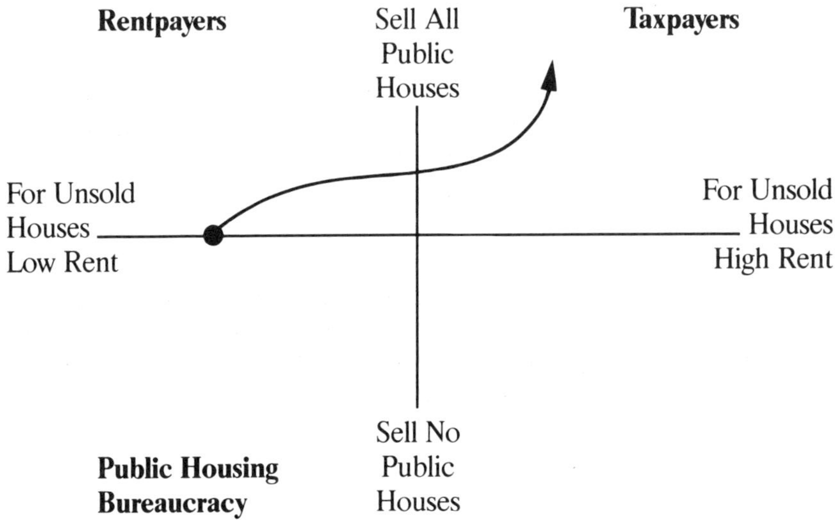

This example illustrates three properties of successful strategies: First, you must create a new issue that was not there before. Second, the new issue must lead to significantly different coalitions than there were before. Third, the process of new coalition formation should be one in which momentum builds over time. In the case of Britain's public housing, as time passes, momentum for the sale of houses builds. The Thatcher government set up the right-to-buy in such a way that the longer a tenant has lived in a public house, the larger the discount is on the purchase price. So with the passage of time, the right-to-buy becomes more and more attractive.

One of the most interesting things about the British experience is that when Margaret Thatcher came into office there was no blueprint to privatize Britain. Privatization was not planned, but dozens of ideas to privatize cropped up all over. It is similar to the invisible hand in economics. A lot of people found it in their self-interest to contribute to the process. With respect to housing, the Thatcher government did not simply announce it was going to sell the houses and then watch people rush out to buy them. The bureaucracy did everything in its power, raised every obstacle that it could raise, to keep people from buying the houses. What made the public-to-private sector transfer of houses work was that people found it in their self-interest to do so. Therefore they used their own resources, their own creativity, their own innovative ability to accomplish it. Privatization in Britain is something that is being felt by literally tens of thousands of people, acting in their own self-interest, much like the invisible hand of economic theory.

Do politicians matter? Yes. In order to set the process in motion, you need a leader—someone who will forge new issues that cause the creation of new coalitions and the disintegration of old coalitions. Leadership is essential. That is why politicians matter, politicians who are receptive to the ideas and institutes that help cause change.

5

Applying the British Model: Case Histories

Stuart Butler

I would like to look at some of the specific opportunities and problems associated with privatization, and to give some hint of the approaches that are necessary in the political context of Washington and around the states. There has been a great deal of thinking by Heritage and other organizations about the fundamental lessons we are learning from Britain, and how to adapt these to the peculiar circumstances of this country.

Differences Between the U.S. and the U.K.

Let me start by noting some of the key differences between privatization in America and privatization in Britain. The first thing to recognize is that when we talk about dismantling in the United States, we primarily are talking about dismantling government services, not selling off assets. While there are in this country extensive holdings of public lands that could be sold to the private sector, we are not really talking about denationalization in the sense that we see in Britain. So, if we are to succeed in using privatization to reduce the size of the U.S. government, we have to find a model that can be applied effectively to human services.

The second point to bear in mind is that the policy-making machine in Washington is very different from that in London. The U.S. has a Congress which is highly sensitive to all kinds of pressure groups, and an Executive Branch that cannot guarantee passage of its proposed legislation. Therefore, it is very difficult in America to put forward a coherent, thought-out plan and move it through Congress with any certainty of the outcome. Thus, we need a model that is flexible and adaptable to the peculiarities of the American political system.

The third point is the need to recognize that in this country legislation moves through Congress because it has the support of very powerful coalitions. Government spending has grown in this country because of coalitions—coalitions of people who are the beneficiaries, administrators and employees of the programs. And a large number of service providers, delivery systems, and contractors gain a great deal from the expansion of government. In other words, there is a very strong private sector lobby working for expansion of the federal government.

The fourth important point is that in this country if you cannot succeed in getting an idea put into place at one level of government, there are other levels to resort to. There are 50 states and the District of Columbia in which to test ideas. This is a very important point that can work to our advantage. Successful privatization in any one of the States or D.C. can serve as an effective demonstration. You do not necessarily have to have the support of Congress. You do not even have to have the initial support of the rest of the country. This is an opportunity that should not be overlooked.

Fifth, an unfortunate fact of life in this country is the central role of the courts and the ease of taking legal action. Because of this, it is sometimes very difficult to move ahead with privatization. Although one talks about assisting the private sector in taking over responsibilities, you have to look over your shoulder very carefully to consider what some U.S. district judge is going to decide. Much of the recent growth of government in this country has been due to decisions made by the judiciary. These decisions simply require changes to take place and programs to be expanded. So we also have to have a model that fits into that reality.

A sixth point to be made with regard to the differences between the U.S. and Britain is the disturbing experience we have had in the U.S. with certain aspects of contracting out as a method of privatization. In many areas contracting out has allowed the private sector to take over responsibility and led to more efficient services, but it also has led to much bigger government. That pushes up total spending, because efficient contractors still push for more contracts. So contracting out can mean that you move from the running of programs by an inefficient bureaucracy to the unleashing of well-organized, highly efficient, lobbying activities by the private sector.

This is clear in the case of defense contracting, where all manner of waste is created and defended by the private sector. In the human services area, it is often overlooked that the vast majority of human services programs are actually delivered by nongovernment providers, primarily nonprofit organizations. I noticed in a recent publication by the Independent Sector, an umbrella organization for many of these nonprofit providers, that they now describe themselves as "Third Party Government." These human service providers are a profession like any other profession, and they have been very effective at building up all kinds of professional licensing barriers to make sure nobody else can provide cheaper services, including people who are true volunteers. Of course, when anybody talks of changing these rules and allowing competition, these professionals come to Washington, dripping with self-righteousness, explaining how standards must be kept up.

Take medical care, for example. We do have a partly privatized medical system in this country. Under our major government health care programs, private providers treat patients and send the bill to Uncle Sam. It is then paid through Medicare and Medicaid. But because of cost-plus reimbursement, there is every incentive for the provider to push costs up. And medical costs in this country have gone up much more rapidly than the general level of inflation.

So, I think contracting out in this country has to be looked at very carefully as an option. Certainly the evidence is very strong that if you go that route you must have effective competition among potential providers. Fortunately, there are some moves now being made in the Reagan Administration to inject competition into contracting out. Still we must be very careful about it. There are plenty of people out there who praise the idea of contracting out so that certain groups in the private sector will be able to use their lobbying power to get more money from the taxpayers.

Building Coalitions

If we are going to move towards privatization in this country we have to bear these realities in mind and begin to look at a general strategy that adapts the concepts of privatization to the U.S. political system. If there is one general conclusion that flows from this, it is the need to build up the same kind of coalitions in the private sector that exist in the public sector—the coalitions that have been responsible for growth of programs. In other words, we need to build coalitions of people who benefit from privatized services, people who can deliver the privatized service, and people who do not quite make it under the existing rules but can be included under the new privatized service. All of these various groups must be employed in building what I call a "mirror image" coalition against the existing coalitions that have been highly effective at maintaining and expanding government programs.

There are ways to strengthen private sector coalitions. One is the use of tax incentives. Highly localized tax incentives can give a distinct advantage to private sector alternatives. Note that there is a very important difference between creating tax advantages which encourage privatization and reducing taxes generally. When you reduce taxes generally, usually nobody gains a great deal. If you localize a tax incentive and concentrate it on people doing things differently—people relying on private rather than public sector services—then you plant firmly in people's minds that they gain a great deal by choosing the private option.

Another method of encouraging strong coalitions for private sector alternatives is to create programs that put financial power in the hands of the beneficiaries of privatization. The voucher, for example, allows you to put in the hands of consumers the right and the financial power to choose. There is no question that if, in the realm of human services, individual beneficiaries were given the financial power to choose among service providers there would be a big shake-up in the way services are provided in this country.

Other Privatization Techniques

Targeting incentives and financial power in such a way that existing coalitions are broken up and new ones are created is very important. It also is crucially important to attack what have been called "barriers to entry"—restrictions that make it difficult for private firms to compete with government. When you have to have a diploma in Early Childhood Psychology to run a private day care center, then private day care becomes very expensive. Unfortunately there has been a lack of action by conservative organizations to expose such restrictive rules. It is said, of course, that somehow these rules are there to protect everybody; this argument has to be exposed. And when you push people proposing absurd rules into court and force them to defend these kinds of restrictions, it becomes much easier to talk about an alternative. At the moment we are not in that position.

It is also possible to use other kinds of measures. At the moment there is a discussion about ways to use antitrust laws to take away the power of cities to restrict competition in all kinds of services. Such action can be used to break up big government and force competition to occur. Historically, the left has been very effective at using the courts and the legal system to promote the growth of big government. But the legal system also can be used to create the opposite effect.

Another, often neglected, area of opportunity is action to alter government funding of academic research. There has been study after study produced by those who want to increase the size of government. A great many of these were funded through government programs. We must inject ourselves into that process and do just the opposite—start cutting off funding for studies that suggest government should be larger, and channeling that money into organizations whose studies propose smaller government.

I recently received a call from an official at HUD interested in ways to privatize housing. This person asked if I knew of anybody who had produced any studies along these lines. He said he had a a list of people who do policy work for the federal government (and he named familiar names), but he did not know anybody else. That just shows you how effective the left has been at building a constituency of researchers who always receive federal grants, who know exactly how to get money, how to produce the results, and then enjoy being treated by the media as producers of "the facts." So changing the research and the funds that support it is very, very important in the long run in breaking up the monolithic view that only government programs are effective.

Another thing we should look at are the rules governing government funding. For example, the federal government must provide money for urban transportation because Congress tells ito. But there is a lot of flexibility under the administrative rule-making process. All kinds of little "riders" can make other things happen as well. We can have rules saying that to have this money, you have to to earmark certain amounts for demonstration projects for private mass transit, for instance. We're not talking about a major shift, just adding things on. In other words, the very thing we've always criticized—the fact that administrators and bureaucrats can formulate rules—means we can reverse policy. We can sow the seeds of the very break-up we're looking for. And we can do this without having a majority in Congress.

The bottom line is to shift the growth of government very slowly and in a gradual way, using the same techniques that have been used to build up government. We want to begin to start moving the other way, and to use many of the methods that have been used by the left very successfully.

In this respect, much can be learned from the British experience. An especially effective technique is to selectively take evidence from abroad and "re-hatch" it to give an image of how things would operate if the same program were put into effect in this country. When the concept of the Enterprise Zone was being promoted in Britain we encouraged people to think of them as tiny Hong Kongs that would be set up all over Britain with absolutely no rules, and with millions of people going to work and prospering. This was important in the very early stages. You have to give a sense of Utopia that is feasible in order to get people to respond. If you discuss things in their grim reality, then you can end up not moving at all.

We still do not have legislation at the federal level to have Enterprise Zones, but we have been very successful around the states. The original enterprise zone idea was to set up demonstration projects to allow for different kinds of economic organization. Proponents said, "Let's have a Socialist Workers' Enterprise Zone over here, and a Free Enterprise Zone over there, and compare them." That essentially has happened at the state level. Indeed, in California, they passed legislation creating a parallel system in which people can choose between a zone with more government and more rules, or one which consists of substantially less. The situation in California gives people the opportunity to compare results, so the demonstration approach is moving forward.

Demonstration projects also create a sort of "trickle up" pressure on Congress to move forward. Thanks to demonstration projects at the state level, even Democrat candidates today are coming out in favor of Enterprise Zones.

Another point to bear in mind is the idea of crafting new constituencies for privatization. There are all kinds of organizations out there that can be very effective in moving the privatization concept forward. Public housing in this country is a good example. The strongest supporters of privatizing public housing in this country are the residents of inner-city projects. These are the people who in the 1960s were thought of as being the radical liberals—the radical community organizers who wanted big government. Yet these are the same people now clamoring to have the government off their backs so they can control what is going on in their community. We have discovered that in moving these ideas forward we can get remarkable support among all kinds of constituents who had been written off by most conservatives. This shows how you can build constituencies that have been long neglected.

The "buyout" is another important technique. If you try to take on an entire constituency that benefits from a federal program, usually you will get clobbered. Any talk about changing Social Security, for instance, has every mother and grandmother up in arms against you. Any talk about selling public lands in this country also has every nature lover against you. But if you begin to recognize that these coalitions have very distinct constituencies within them, with very different reasons for supporting the programs, then you can begin to look for ways of buying out constituent elements and breaking up the coalitions.

In the case of public lands, for example, there has been a proposal put forward by economists John Baden and Richard Stroup in Montana. One of the biggest problems, they note, is that everyone thinks if we sell public land we are going to give away wilderness areas and the fish and wildlife will be plundered. Baden and Stroup proposed that since the conservationist organizations are so concerned, we ought to *give* them these areas. In fact, the National Audubon Society already owns parts of very sensitive wildlife areas, and they have oil companies on these lands. The oil company operations are carefully monitored, and the Audubon Society gets revenue from them with which it buys other lands. Once they get ownership, in other words, the conservationist organizations begin to make rational decisions about how the land should be managed. If they don't have control of the land, their incentive is to push as hard as possible to stop anything happening within these areas.

Social Security is another area with various constituencies. By default, the president has done us a favor by saying he is not going to touch benefits for people now retired or anyone nearing retirement. Now we can remove benefit cuts from the discussion, and concentrate on the real problem—the problems facing future generations—without threatening elderly voters.

Breaking up constituencies in this way is critically important. It is fruitless to attack the welfare budget by saying, "How can we stop this inner-city kid from getting food stamps? How can we cut him off?" You don't get anywhere in this country by doing that.

A final point to bear in mind, especially in sensitive areas like Social Security, is that you cannot be successful at making a change until you have created an alternative people can understand and become used to. So when talking about privatization, the first step must be to build a parallel system that does not challenge in any way the program already in existence. Direct attacks can come later, when you have something in place that people know about. In the case of Social Security, the first step is to build a completely private parallel system. We should talk in terms of the parallel system strengthening Social Security and adding to it. We should not attack Social Security, rather we should talk about a public/private partnership. In this way it does not frighten anybody. Later on we can start looking at ways to make the alternative more attractive to people. This is the key to tackling human services. There has been a failure by the budget cutters to identify the alternatives, to strengthen them, and then to politicize them. Give the people an alternative to embrace before you start attacking the system currently in existence.

Today the U.S. may well be in a situation similar to Margaret Thatcher's in 1980. The Reagan Administration has used traditional conservative measures to try to deal with the budget. Yet the budget has grown steadily ever since Reagan took office; the administration has been totally unsuccessful at reducing government spending. Now there is a sense of exhaustion in the administration and Congress. They are beginning to say, "There must be some other technique that we can use to deal with this problem." So we have a golden opportunity to start putting forth the idea of privatization as a decisive strategy to change the nation's political dynamics.

6

Building New Coalitions as a Key to Privatization

Fred L. Smith

Special interest groups come to Washington for special favors for the same reason Willie Sutton went to the bank — it is where the money is! Willie probably doubted the morality of stealing, but he found that crime paid. In a similar way, special interest groups are not evil, but their work pays. To change public policy, we must raise the cost of raiding the public treasury. Special interest groups will come to Washington as long as it advances their interests, and we must change that.

In order to accomplish this change we need to build coalitions. Coalitions bridge the gap between ideas and public policy. All of us believe that ideas have consequences. But ideas need champions; they do not walk out of journals or analytic textbooks on their own. They have to be carried into battle. Coalitions can help determine whether ideas are advanced or not.

What I mean by coalitions is a broad kind of advocacy group, an ad hoc group of individuals and organizations who join together for a specific, targeted purpose. This produces a kind of rifle-shot approach to defeating or supporting a specific issue. In our initial stages the approach should be aimed toward defeating legislation that further restricts economic freedom. As we become a more powerful force, we will then be in a stronger position to get legislation passed.

Successful coalitions involve four sub-tasks. First, there is the analytical task which is critical. Fact sheets must be prepared. Data analysis must be conducted. Where possible, the analysis should point to successful examples from other countries. Almost every attempt at deregulation has started with questions such as, "What is happening in Australia?"or "What are the Canadians doing?"or "What are the Swedes doing?" The success stories from "over there" can provide clear examples that make it easier to have particular policies or approaches considered seriously.

This approach is nothing new. The liberal/left has been using this technique for many, many years. Remember, they went to Russia and announced that the future worked! I am hopeful that we would not make this type of mistake, that we instead will show there are areas where deregulation can work, where free markets can, in fact, provide better ways to provide services.

Second, we need outreach efforts. We need to pull in our natural and sometimes our not-so-natural allies. They can be very effective in promoting our policies, particularly with liberal groups. And if they are working with us, they are staying out of the areas where they can do a lot of harm. We certainly need them. We are not going to win this alone.

Third, media relations are becoming increasingly important. We have got to get our message out to a lot of people. On any given issue, the public needs to be informed; their fears about possible negative effects need to be addressed. On the issue of Social Security, for example, we have to convince people that we are not going to cut off their retirement income. On the issue of the Rural Electric Administration, we have to let people know we are not going to cut the lights off in rural America. This means we have to reach a lot of outlets in a lot of places in order to communicate effectively. It also means we have to have good hard facts and arguments to convince people.

Fourth, we need to lobby. Lobbying is an activity in which most conservative groups have not been heavily involved compared to the traditional liberal public interest groups. Although it is not now a major part of our activities, in the future we have to expand these efforts to persuade legislators to take the right stands on the policy issues.

In a successful coalition a large number of organizations come together to focus on one particular issue. These organizations may include some that do not usually agree on much of anything except on the specific issue. In joining an umbrella group that focuses on that issue, they agree to put aside all other disagreements.

I would like to discuss two examples of coalitions in which I was actively involved, draw some lessons from those experiences, and give examples of areas where I think we are now ripe for new coalitions—areas where we can change the public policy agenda. The two case histories are the Clinch River Breeder Reactor Project and funding for the International Monetary Fund.

The Breeder Reactor Project was started in the early 1970s using government subsidies to commercialize energy development processes. It was believed at the time that we were running out of uranium and nobody in the market had noticed. Thus, it was argued, government aid was required. The initial opposition to the project came largely from anti-nuclear goups, who gained a certain amount of success but could not stop the project. So they asked for help; they went out and tried to get allies. They went to the National Taxpayers' Union and the Council for a Competitive Economy and asked them to get involved.

We said we opposed the breeder reactor project but not on their terms. Our position was that every energy source should pay its own way, and that government should not be subsidizing one energy source to give it an advantage over others. This position, based on economic grounds, also offered a more persuasive case and made it possible to bring in conservative support. The final victory in this case (funding for the project was defeated) came with a tremendous amount of support from traditional conservatives, both in the House and in the Senate. The efforts of Senator Gordon Humphrey (R.-N.H.) were especially critical to the project's defeat in the Senate.

The factual case for our position was well documented. We always were able to produce the right analysis at the right time. It is critical to anticipate what arguments will be raised and to be ready with a immediate response. In this situation, the proponents of the project pointed to foreign examples: They said that a German project was working, as well as another project in Japan. It is not easy to find out the facts of such cases, but it is essential because there is always the argument from the other side that, "Sure it is not working right now, but we will get more money, a wiser management and then it will work!" This argument is made especially forcefully if there is a lot of money at stake.

Our coalition worked to reframe the issue, and by the time the effort succeeded the coalition included liberals, church groups, the "good government" types, and, most significantly, social conservatives. When the last vote on the issue came up in the Senate, proponents of the project had 48 votes, and had always been able to squeeze out the one or two more votes that were needed. But some of the Senate's social conservatives came out in opposition very strongly at the end, taking the position of opposing corporate welfare when it came at the expense of social welfare. This populist approach resulted in the defeat of the Breeder Reactor Project.

The International Monetary Fund issue was quite different, and was a much easier issue for conservatives to win. Many conservative groups are opposed to foreign aid, and since the IMF funding question can be viewed as a foreign-aid issue, their opposition to increased funding for the IMF was easier to generate. The International Monetary Fund is a means whereby creditor nations provide debtor nations with the funds they need to repay their debts. It is a way of ensuring that the nations that have wasted their resources are buffered from the consequences of their actions. It is a kind of an international loan guarantee program—foreign aid from one government to another government.

We had an interesting group of conservatives working on the issue. We also were trying to make overtures to the liberal groups. Foreign aid has long had a tremendous support base in the liberal community, but there have been some recent defections. For example, some of the church groups are beginning to question, at long last, whether aid money is really getting positive results. In addition, some environmentalists finally have begun to understand the lesson that good economics also is good environmentalism; that, in effect, many foreign aid programs involve exporting the Corps of Engineers mentality to the Third World. Thankfully they are beginning to oppose this.

Some business groups also got involved in the IMF issue. An interesting situation caused the copper industry in the U.S. to join. Many Third World countries have copper industries, often these are state-owned enterprises, and when they get into trouble the country's economy is affected. Then the IMF comes in. It says, "You're in trouble. You have got to improve your situation. We want you to export more and deflate your currencies." So they deflate their currencies, which lowers the relative cost of export products as opposed to import products. Resources flow into the only thing they have to export—copper. They start pouring copper into the world market, and the price of copper drops. All of which, of course, is natural and expected.

However, the IMF also is set up to basically ensure that the Third World is protected in these situations. So we have a situation where one arm of the IMF drives down the price of copper and another arm of the IMF drives the price of copper back up. That means that the copper-exporting countries like Chile are in good shape. But it also means that the U.S. copper industry has to face a low world price, while the taxes it pays go toward helping subsidize the exports of their competitors. That is why the U.S. copper industry joined us.

The final vote on this issue was in the House. There was about a seven-vote difference, the closest the IMF ever came to losing funding. We are now in the second round of that fight. There will be a third and a fourth, and so on. A coalition effort need not be a one-shot affair. It may be a multi-battle war. You almost never win the the first battle, but as time passes, you build support.

Earlier, I pointed out the sub-tasks involved in a successful coalition effort. I now would like to assess how well market-oriented groups are doing and where improvement is needed in these efforts.

The best thing we have going for us these days is very high-quality public policy analysis. The American Enterprise Institute, the Hoover Institute, the National Center for Policy Analysis—these think tanks are prepared and increasingly able to turn out a special piece of work on a targeted issue. Our competency and our ability to relate to practical political battles has improved dramatically.

In media relations I think the picture is still mixed. The media still seems to believe that more government regulation promotes the public interest. Market approaches are suspect; they are perceived by the media as promoting efficiency but being uncompassionate and uncaring. We do best when we can frame our ideas in liberal terms, when we "out bleed" the bleeding hearts. We do a much better job when we can talk about helping the poor.

In outreach efforts, I don't think conservatives are as effective at networking and building good bridges to the other side as liberal groups have been. The traditional "public interest" groups are more effective. Because many groups often contact each other regularly, they are much more able and willing to cooperate in short-term working relationships. They often call each other to get signatures on a letter. It would require us meeting for several weeks before we could agree on the terms under which we would write a common letter. As we work together longer, as more and more conservative groups begin to know each other's agendas better, undoubtedly we will become more effective at cooperating.

It also takes a long time for many issues to jell, and it often has been difficult for our side to develop a continuity on certain issues. There is a tendency for our side still to address an issue on a short-term basis—through press releases, a monograph, a report—rather than a continual tracking, day-in and day-out through low times and high times, always trying to know in advance what issue is coming up.

Coalitions also require credibility. You cannot be a front group for industry or any other special interest. You have to be perceived as saying something you really believe is true. You can be ideological, but you cannot be perceived as being bought. One of the problems that conservative free-market groups face is that because our rhetoric is free-enterprise and limited government, and because many special interest groups use the same rhetoric, our views are mistaken by the press. That is a danger we must avoid. It means we have to have a different strategy than liberal political groups. They can take a narrow stand on a narrow issue, such as access for the handicapped in downtown Washington, and be listened to and be perceived as a credible organization because they are not linked to any special interest group.However, because a market-oriented group may take a position in support of industry's view, we are more likely to be perceived as being nothing more than a front for a special interest.

One way to deal with this problem is by being consistent. We must be consistent in dealing with a whole range of issues. If, for example, we are going to advocate financial institution deregulation, we probably should be willing to oppose the International Monetary Fund. Our principles have to be consistent over a broad range of areas.

We also have to be more willing to cooperate in coalitions comparable to the public interest coalitions on the liberal side. One reason coalitions produce results is that when lawmakers realize that many different groups spanning the ideological horizon are in support of a position, they feel safe sticking their necks out.

There is a big difference between this kind of activist coalition and traditional public policy research. Research papers are written based on an expectation about the timing and the content of a public policy debate. However, Congress can be very unpredictable. Something happens, and all of a sudden an issue that was expected to come up is forced off the schedule. You already have sent your research in, the paper has gone to a staff member and is buried under a pile of reading material. The issue then comes up one month, two months, or six months later. The staff person does not have time to dig it out again, and your analysis does not get read because it was not there at the right time. You have to be aware always that the analysis must be ready and available at the precise time the issue comes up again. And you have to know when that time is.

There is also a tremendous need for good interpersonal skills in coalition building. I know that the political process is a new area for us. This is because we first had to develop the intellectual ammunition to fight the battles. Ten years ago there were not many of us fighting. We had our original thinkers, but we did not have think tanks. We do now. The next step is to move into the implementation process. I think we wrongly thought that other people automatically would see the worth of our positions and take up the implementation process.

In this country, politicians tend to accept the political landscape; they do not move the trees around very much. We have to restructure the political landscape, then the politicans will go along with our ideas. They do not have the time and the courage required to do a lot of restructuring themselves.

Similarly, business groups are forced to take tactical stands. They do not have the freedom or the stability to lose as many times as we can. We can take a long-term position. What is good for General Motors may be good for the U.S. economy or the U.S. consumer. But a General Motors' spokesman cannot say that in public any longer. He ends up in trouble if he tries. Other people have to do it.

There are whole range of issues on the horizon that offer a tremendous opportunity for coalition building. We need to take our messages and build coalitions around them. We have the right ideas; we have got the right principles. The evidence suggests we can win.

7

Privatization From the Bottom Up

Robert Poole

For many years I have viewed privatization as perhaps the most important single issue in advancing the cause of limited government, and of shrinking the bloated governments we have at all levels—local, state and federal. The reason for that is a point made by several other speakers—namely the tremendous persuasive power of real, live examples, in contrast to theoretical arguments.

The happy fact is we have hundreds if not thousands of real-world examples of privatization. These are very effective weapons, if we look hard enough for them and dramatize them to people. You can talk yourself blue in the face and have wonderful studies to show why private, competitive enterprise does a better and cheaper job than monopolistic government bureaus. But seeing private fire engines running up and down your street, seeing the crews putting out fires, seeing them do it successfully at a demonstrably lower cost, persuades people far more effectively than any journal articles you can come up with.

The responsibility of the Reason Foundation is to find and publicize examples of privatization for their teaching value. Our goal is to debunk the idea of the government as the only service provider, and as the solver of social problems. Two of our program areas share the burden of advancing privatization. One is *Reason* magazine, a monthly magazine on current affairs that is out there in the intellectual marketplace competing with the *New Republic*, *National Review*, *Nation*, *Harper's*, and other publications. The other is our think tank called The Local Government Center.

Reason uses feature articles that take a specific example of privatization and make it real to people. We talk about the real, live human beings providing a service or performing a function. We talk about how it works as a competitive market instead of a monopoly. We do what 60 Minutes and ABC's 20/20 program do—dramatize with real people what privatization is like.

Privatization Success Stories: Private Streets

Although libertarians often are portrayed as crazy people who want to sell the streets, we actually have found private streets, in fact some very dramatic examples of them. One particularly interesting example is in St. Louis, where there are hundreds of city blocks in residential areas that had been turned over to neighborhood organizations and made the private property of those people. If you go to St. Louis and wander through the neighborhoods you can see the difference between well-kept middle class streets and, a block or two away, rundown slum-type streets. The variable that makes the difference is private ownership.

Dramatic changes happen when people have gotten together to buy a street from the city, made it a private street, and decided they are going to make it a good, safe place to live. Actual results bear this out. Crime rates are half as much or lower than crime rates on the streets two or three blocks away that are public. Also, property values increase dramatically. We sent a reporter to St. Louis to do the story, and dramatized it with photos and first-person vignettes of families who lived on those streets—what it was like before they formed the association and bought the streets, and how things have changed. That is how we make voluntary, self-help efforts real to people so they can see what is possible and that they do not need to turn to government to improve their lives or their neighborhoods.

Electric Utilities

A reader of *Reason* magazine (and this is where we get many of our story ideas) sent us a newspaper clipping about four years ago saying that some little town somewhere had two power companies providing electricity. We published that in our Trends section and Gordon Tullock wrote in and said, "That is not the only one. There are about 25 or 50 of these around the country." Meanwhile we learned that an economist had adopted this issue as an area to study. So we got in touch with the economist, got all of his papers and dozens of journal articles—ten years' worth of research on this strange phenomenon—and decided to do the story.

We sent a reporter to Lubbock, Texas, a city of about 100,000 people and the largest city with competing electrical companies. She went around and talked to the people who lived in the neighborhoods and took photographs of two sets of power lines. There were no more poles than there were in other neighborhoods where there are lines for telephones, cable television, and so forth. They had doubled up so it was no more unsightly than in other communities.

Our reporter did a fantastic story that showed how consumers were much better served by competition. The economist's studies showed that the rates were lower in towns with competing electric power. He stood the conventional public utility theory on its head, because traditional theory says it is natural for the cost to be higher with competition because of duplication of facilities, neglecting any effect on improving efficiency due to competition. The fact of the matter is that in Lubbock consumers can switch, on three days' notice, from one power company to another any time they are dissatisfied with the service. And you had better believe that the people there are enthusiastic! That story went on to win the John Hancock Award for Excellence in 1982.

The Privatization Data Base

Journalism alone is often not sufficient to sell privatization, especially to the people in local government who have to make decisions subject to all of the pressure groups within their own bureaucracy. These include the public employee unions, who resist change and fight tooth and nail against privatization because it usually means becoming more efficient by paying only the number of people needed to do the job. So you automatically are up against a strong opposition. We decided we needed a lot more specialized material to fight these battles—the instances when taxpayers or enlightened city officials want to privatize services and need specific help. We went to work exploring ways to fill this need.

It is interesting how events in different countries reinforce one another. In 1979, I wrote a book called *Cutting Back City Hall*, which documented the extent of privatization across the United States. The book referred to privatization studies such as E.S. Savas' study on garbage collection. The book was picked up in England by the Adam Smith Institute, which popularized many of its case studies and started the privatization ball rolling in a very organized way in England. Later, Steve Savas went to work for HUD and organized a privatization roundtable discussion at which Madsen Pirie explained the role of the Adam Smith Institute in providing information to further the cause of privatization in England. And all of a sudden I realized, "My gosh, that is the kind of thing *we* should be doing!" And so the circle came back around; we decided what the Reason Foundation should do is start providing much more specific, targeted information to assist local governments with privatization, which is what we subsequently have done.

Now we already had created the Local Government Center as a subsidiary and began publishing a newsletter called Fiscal Watchdog, which is targeted primarily to local government decision-makers, local chambers of commerce, and local taxpayer organizations. It is a monthly newsletter, now six years old, that reports on ongoing developments in privatizataion—which cities have done what, what new studies are out—giving a continuous supply of ammunition about actual, practical examples and studies that can be very useful.

Yet we found that people called us and wanted more. For example, a city official would call from Iowa and say, "We are thinking about contracting out street sweeping in our city. Can you tell me if any other city in Iowa is doing this?" Well, how on earth would we know?!

Fortunately, HUD came to the rescue again. One of the projects that Steve Savas initiated while he was at HUD was to have the International City Management Association do a nationwide survey on all kinds of alternative service delivery methods, including contracting out, vouchers, and franchises. The data from that became available to us last year. A donor supplied a microcomputer, and we have spent most of this past year developing a data base listing all of the thousands of examples of privatization that were included in this nationwide survey, plus everything that we had accumulated in our files over the last five or six years.

It is now possible for anyone in the United States who has a specific question about the extent of privatization in nearly 70 different public services in any part of the United States to come to us and, for a very modest charge, get a printout showing which specific communities are privatizing and in which areas. They then can contact the city managers or mayors in those communities and find out what the problems are, who the contractors are and other information.

The Local Government Center also is going to be very useful in dealing with the needs of local officials and taxpayer groups who want to promote privatization, and who want to respond to opposition arguments such as, "This is something with which there has been very little experience," "It is a risky thing to do," and "It has never been tried." These arguments are not true, but hardly anyone knows it.

What kind of results come from providing this sort of information? Well, we get inquiries all the time from local officials and the press. We get invited to speak at conferences and before groups such as the International City Management Association and the National Association of Regional Councils. We currently are assisting the Chamber of Commerce in Philadelphia and several other cities with ideas about good things to try to privatize in their cities. And we get articles in various newspapers and magazines on a fairly regular basis. Those of you who see *Venture* magazine may have noticed a cover story on privatization in July, 1984.

Entrepreneurs of Privatization

Privatization creates entrepreneurial opportunities in many specific business areas—air traffic control and fire protection for example. In these areas, entrepreneurs have started companies and found a market, and we hope these early successes will encourage other companies to go into business. I want to take just a few minutes to describe these areas of privatization that we have worked on, and to trace how one thing has led to another and what the future prospects may be.

Private Fire Departments

This case study is very unusual. It is a difficult area to privatize because people see anything involving public safety as somehow inherently more governmental than is picking up garbage or delivering a similar service. Nevertheless, there are in Europe and the United States various private enterprise fire departments that operate and do a tremendous job.

Reason was the first national publication to do a journalistic account of a private fire department. We looked at the one in Scottsdale, Arizona. About a year and a half after we did that it was picked up on CBS' 60 Minutes; *Reason* was the primary source for that. But, that was not the end of the story by any means. As a result of the 60 Minutes program, several entrepreneurs, people who had some experience either as firefighters or as dealers in fire equipment, were inspired to start their own companies in different parts of the country. I know of three—one in Georgia, one in Illinois, and one in Oregon—that were inspired directly by watching that broadcast. They formed companies, have gone after business, and have succeeded in being in the private sector fire business.

About two years ago, a group of these people who had been corresponding and comparing notes decided to form a trade association. Today we have the Private Sector Fire Association, which has eight companies as members. It has produced a very useful 20-page question-and-answer brochure designed to answer all of the "red herring" charges that fire unions raise whenever anyone proposes privatizing fire service. In addition, they have produced model specifications that any community can use when asking for bids for fire services. They hold twice-a-year gatherings at the same time the International Association of Fire Chiefs holds a convention. They hold a convention in an adjacent room in the same hotel—a rump session! I have been to several of these meetings.

Reason has continued to follow up on the growth of this industry. We did a couple of stories in 1983. One was on the development of two competing private enterprise fire companies in Oregon. The result of that competition was that the cost of fire protection went down and the quality went up, and both are still in business. Another story was about two very bitter battles in New England where cities attempted to contract out fire protection. The labor unions brought in resources from their national offices and waged an all-out dirty campaign. In both cases, the unions won.

The story about Oregon was picked up in an article in Newsweek in April of 1983. This, in turn, was one of the factors leading ABC News to do a three-part series on privatization of city services. Another result of these events was that the first national convention on private sector fire service was held in December, 1983, in Orlando, Florida, and I was invited to give the lead-off presentation. That, in turn, led to other developments. The editor of *International Fire Chief* magazine attended the conference and devoted a special issue to four articles on "Private Fire Services: Threat or Promise?" The articles gave a very fair presentation of the case for private fire-fighting, and the extent to which it has been growing.

Recently I attended the latest convention of the Private Sector Fire Association. The grim news is there has not been a single new case of a city deciding to contract out fire protection in 1984, although there have been a number of battles over it. The firefighters' union is pouring tremendous resources into these battles. The private companies, coming from Florida or Arizona, do not know the local community, do not know how it works, and have to spend a lot of time putting people up in hotel rooms while they are fighting the battle. In every case this year the private companies have lost. So this may not be one of the best growth areas for privatization, but it has been a tremendously important educational one because it gets people's attention. It is startling. It is unusual. If fire protection can be privatized, well, practically anything can be. It has had a great deal of teaching value, even if it has not been a very good area to invest in if you are an entrepreneur or an investor.

Private Air Traffic Control

This is another interesting case history of the evolution of an industry. About four years ago, we did a book at the Reason Foundation called *Instead of Regulation: Alternatives to Federal Regulatory Agencies.* In one chapter I suggested that, based on evidence from overseas, air traffic control is basically just a business. It can be paid for by the users, and it ought to be turned over to private enterprise in this country instead of having the Federal Aviation Administration providing that service out of tax money.

Well, during the second week of the air traffic controllers' strike, I got a call from John McClaughry on the White House staff saying, "Didn't I read somewhere that you have proposed privatization of air traffic controllers?" So they flew me to Washington to brief the head of the FAA and the Secretary of Transportation. I had to cobble together on the plane and in the hotel room a specific plan for how it could be achieved, which I had not done in the chapter. I had only used illustrations from overseas. But I devised what seemed to be a very workable plan that dealt with the danger of strikes by private controllers who could potentially shut down the whole country. I think I came up with a unique solution that deals with the problems in an effective way.

Unfortunately, the head of the FAA at the time, Lynn Helms, wanted absolutely no part of this threat to his bureaucratic empire, and managed to torpedo it. The strike got settled by firing the strikers and the whole thing died down. I was not really satisfied with that quick defeat on the issue. I thought that perhaps if we had been better prepared we might have been able to seize that window of opportunity.

In any event, since it was going to take a long time to rebuild the air traffic control system, we started talking to Stuart Butler and Fred Smith here in Washington about what could be done to move this issue along. We tried to see if there was a way to build support for it.

Early in 1983 the three of us went around to various Congressional committees that deal with aviation, briefed them on what we had learned so far, and tried to find out what it would take to build political support for privatized air traffic control. We said, "What would you need as evidence? And they said, "Well, the best thing we need is practical evidence showing" how this works. Do you have examples?" We knew there already were private companies running control towers at small airports in this country. So we dispatched John Doherty, a writer and an airline pilot, to do a journalistic story about how these companies do it. That was published in *Reason* in May of 1983.

It turned out to be a fantastic case study. Private air traffic controllers can do it for less than half the cost. They do an excellent job because they are much more efficient. There is a track record of about eight firms in the business already. We also learned that the FAA just recently had started contracting out on a very modest scale—three control towers they were in the process of reopening as they rebuilt from the strike. They had new legislative authority to do that.

What happened was that the American Association of Airport Executives got copies of that article and sent them all over the world to practically everybody they could think of. Being the trade association for small airports, they really liked the idea of getting out from under the FAA and having the contract program greatly expanded so more of their airports could have control towers. That led to FAA hearings at which Fred Smith and John Doherty testified in August of '83, and that in turn led to expansion of the contract tower program. The growing visibility of this led to NBC's Today Show to do a very favorable five minutes on the privatization of control towers in the spring of '84.

More recently, Fred Smith and I have been trying to raise the issue as part of the solution for coping with the tremendous problems the air traffic control system is having, including not enough capacity due to growth of the economy and to greatly expanded air travel because of airline deregulation. There also is a big problem due to lack of market pricing at airports. We are trying to push a combined solution of contracting out air traffic control operations (which would enable private companies to hire experienced controllers the federal government cannot rehire) and market pricing to deal with the airport congestion.

Picking Issues

This is a very live issue. It is one where we may see some real progress if we can build the kind of coalition that we have talked about. I think we can draw some important lessons from these experiences. We need to pick our issues carefully, since some are easier than others. There are areas such as fire protection that may have great teaching value, but they are very difficult to make progress in because of the special interest groups involved and the incentives they face. If we are to make real breakthroughs in building industries that take large amounts of business away from government, we need to first focus on the ones we have the best chance of winning.

8

Privatization From the Top Down and From the Outside In

E.S. Savas

I have been asked to describe my experiences in introducing privatization from the top down, and to distill those experiences into some rules for action. Then I will describe some of the things I would like to see happen over the next several years. My emphasis will be on local government, because in the United States 80 percent of all government employees work for state or local governments. We speak of "large government," and yes, the federal budget is large, but if one measures government by the number of employees, it is state and local government that is larger. This is truly an area with extraordinary opportunities for privatization.

I would like to begin with the New York City government. When I was First Deputy Administrator of New York under Mayor John Lindsay, I one day found myself involved in a disastrous snow storm. This snow storm was ultimately what got me started in privatization. The snow was not cleaned up for more than a week, a failure which created a significant political problem. The city had done a poor job, and the mayor asked me to find out what had happened and what could be done to prevent it from ever happening again. I discovered that in the midst of a snow emergency, when the department responsible for cleaning up after the storm was operating under emergency conditions (working overtime) the men were plowing and sanding only about 50 percent of the time. The rest of the time was consumed in breaks—warmup breaks, coffee breaks, lunch breaks, wash breaks, fueling breaks, and so on. And I thought, "Gee, if this is how the department works in an emergency, I wonder how it works when it is not an emergency."

That was the New York City Department of Sanitation, and its main activity throughout the year is collecting solid waste. So I started an in-house study of the department, and compared it with the private sector. We found that private firms were able to collect solid waste for about $19 per ton, whereas the NYC Department of Sanitation cost $49 per ton—a ratio of 2.6 to 1. We then examined other services. In street repair, we found that the ratio also was 2.6 to l. About that time I met Madsen Pirie, who dubbed this figure "Savas' Law." He has published various things about this fixed ratio, which may be the Planck's constant of privatization.

There was a lot of publicity about our findings—front-page stories, radio, television debates, and the usual hoopla. There also was a nice media battle between myself and the Sanitation Commissioner. I advocated contracting out a small portion of his department's activities to see what would happen, and he was protecting his bloated bureaucracy.

In fact, because of the political strength of the affected union, nothing was done about the suggestion in New York at that time. But the seeds had been planted. Good government groups picked up the privatization idea, and because New York is a media capital there was a lot of attention given to this issue. The idea of contracting out services expanded to a national scale. That was the first stage.

The second stage of the story of top-down privatization occurred from a university base, when I organized and directed a large project on privatization funded by the National Science Foundation. God bless that particular government agency, because with a $2 million budget, we were able to look very systematically and carefully at the whole issue of contracting out. The project from beginning to end took about five years. The results were convincing, unassailable, and irrefutable. As a matter of fact, the nationwide union that represented state and local government workers tried very hard to kill that project while we were in the middle of it; they tried to exercise political pressure through Congress to stop the funding for the project. But to the National Science Foundation's credit, it did not give in.

Now we get to stage three. Stage three was the exploitation of these findings by industry. There is a well-established, private solid waste industry that reaches every hamlet in America. Here was a large, nationwide army ready to utilize these research findings, and to bring the word to every town and village in America. And that is what it did. The trade association of the industry took our report, distilled information from it, ran ads in various trade magazines about the findings, and engaged in a great deal of publicity and salesmanship across the country. At the same time we were describing our results to the media, to mayors and city officials, and to any group of three or more who would listen.

The results were striking. After only six years, there was an increase of 50 percent in the number of cities in the United States that were contracting out solid waste collection. This was a successful, industrywide and nationwide example of privatization that started as a top-down effort, and became an all-around effort. It also can be described as having taken place from the outside in, rather than from the inside out, inasmuch as I was an outsider in this field.

It was very gratifying earlier this year, when I was addressing a group of mayors in the Pacific Northwest, to discover that public officials now realize that the private sector can do it better than the public sector. That is an extraordinary acknowledgement coming from public officials. The issues that remain for them are when to do it, how to do it, political obstacles, and the human problems of the labor force. The argument as to who can do it better and why has finally been won.

What general rules or techniques can be identified here? Let me resort to a farm analogy. There are four rules to good farming:

- Choose fertile soil;

- Plant the seeds;

- Fertilize;

- Propagate.

What do I mean by "choose fertile soil"? I mean choose it ideally. Choose areas where there are industry salesmen who can take your products, disseminate them, and sell them. That is fertile soil. All it needs is spade work for coalition building. In other words, the ideal setting is where there are immediate beneficiaries who can benefit in the short-term from privatization.

The second step is planting seeds. It is not very important whether it is done by ideological means or other means. The important thing is to get the word out, to disseminate the virtues and the advantages of privatization. In my own view I think the ideological approach is useful among ourselves, among converts, but it is less useful to the outside world. We have to package our products differently to reach different groups. It is like a seed catalog with dozens of choices.

The third step is to fertilize. I mean fertilize with facts, not with manure. (There is a fair amount of manure in this field, and for that matter in all fields involving the public sector.) Hard, substantiated facts are absolutely mandatory. We cannot "wing-and-prayer" it. We need a firm foundation to build on so we can persuade people authoritatively and knowledgeably.

The fourth step is to propagate. It is important to propagate pragmatically, and package our product prudently. The word "privatization" actually is an impediment to success in most cases, although it is a very convenient shorthand term among ourselves. But in the world at large, people do not really understand it; however, if you say you can do it better and cheaper, they will understand. I think the best approach is to stress better service at a lower cost. In trying to promote greater use of the private sector among federal agencies, we are not using the word "privatization." We simply are saying that it is a productivity enhancement measure—we are enhancing productivity by introducing competition.

I would like to go back to the delightful phrase that Eamonn Butler used, "There is no point in trying to persuade turkeys of the virtues of an early Thanksgiving." We are promoting a major change in the way government does its business, and there is no point in coming at people ideologically and with a club. What I have found effective in dealing with public officials is to explain that what I am really talking about is job enhancement. I do not tell them they should be out of business or that I want to abolish their responsibilities. The approach that I have taken is to say, "Look, right now you are conceiving your role as commissioner of parks as running a department that mows the grass and prunes the trees. You should expand the vision of your job and think of it as being responsible for making sure that the grass and the trees are well maintained.

Once you take that step you will find yourself in the position of a manufacturer who has a make-or-buy decision. If you are manufacturing automobiles, do you buy the headlights or do you make the headlights in-house? Do you buy from an outside supplier, or do you produce them with your own labor?"

Public officials should be in that same kind of position. They can make a decision about buying the service from the outside or producing it in-house. It is all part of their responsibility to look at their jobs in this way. This is a more effective approach than the negative argument I have heard too often that implies people who work in government are inferior to those who work in the private sector. That is not the case at all. In fact, management in government is a much more difficult task. Because of bureaucracy, the system conspires to make public services less efficient and less effective than privately provided services.

Another point is that we privatizers have full-product lines. We have lots of seeds in our catalog. We not only have free-market arrangements to offer, we can offer choice among free-market arrangements. There are some services that cannot be subjected immediately to a free-market solution, and never will. But if we cannot sell one free-market arrangement we can turn the pages of the seed catalog and try to sell something else. We can try to sell volunteer organizations, for example, as a mechanism for delivering certain municipal services. A community can levy a special tax or it can enlist volunteer services to provide fire protection, safety patrols, ambulance service, and many other kinds of services. There are many communities—even communities within New York City—that do this sort of thing.

Turn the page again. If you cannot sell free-market arrangements, and you cannot sell a volunteer arrangement for providing a local service, turn the page and sell something else. Sell franchising. Sell vouchers. They are on the next page. We all know the virtures of vouchers, particularly for schools, but if you cannot sell vouchers, sell contracting out. There are many examples in the United States of contracting out of public education. Whenever a community is too small to support its own school and buys educational services from the school in the next district, that is contracting out. In the community I live in, parents from nearby towns can choose not to send their children to the local public school, and can instead send them to the public school in my community. In this case the parents pay individually. If the town sends a whole group of students, then it is paid for by the town, one contracting with the other. In Minnesota some schools are buying art courses from a private group of art teachers.

To continue with the catalog, and to reinforce the point, if you have got a lot of products to offer and if one will not work, there is always another. It is important to recognize that we do have a full-product line. Don't stick with just one product that may not serve all purposes on all occasions at all times.

I would like to refer briefly to another example of privatizing from the top down. This experience came when I served in the U.S. Department of Housing and Urban Development during the first two years of the Reagan Administration, as Assistant Secretary for Policy Development and Research. One of my main policy thrusts was vouchers for public housing.

We inherited a program where the principal means of providing housing assistance to low-income Americans was either through public housing (which involves creating public housing bureaucracies and all the attendant ills), or through giving money to private builders to build houses. Either way, the houses essentially were labeled, "This building is for poor people only." That was how we provided housing assistance to low-income households. And yet, lying right at hand with $150 million worth of completed research was the voucher system. Using housing vouchers instead of subsidized construction, we could house almost three times more people with the same amount of money. The average family being assisted by new construction programs was getting a monthly subsidy from the American public of $415. In California, the average subsidy for newly-constructed housing assistance was $915 a month! There had to be a better way.

After some small battles, vouchers were adopted as Administration policy. But the Congress was very resistant, even though all of the evidence showed that not only could you house more people for the same amount of money, but you could provide people with choice and dignity. Low-income people would not be forced to live in houses labeled "for the poor only." Oddly enough, Congress was very resistant to this notion. The reason seems to be that builders make larger campaign contributions than poor people do. In any event, at long last in 1984, Congress grudgingly agreed not to build much more new housing and finally authorized a demonstration program, even though in the 1970s we already had spent $150 million on successful demonstrations of vouchers. This, too, must be judged a successful instance of privatization from the top down.

Although many people ultimately contributed to the effort, I take some personal pride in seeing the HUD budget decline from about $32 billion a year to about $14 billion a year, in the span of four years.

What is next? What might be done over the next several years to enhance and promote the concept of privatization? I would like to see a White House conference on privatization. Early in his first term Reagan created the President's Task Force on Private Sector Initiatives. It is an organization with a very broad agenda, looking at a variety of ways the private sector can be utilized to achieve public purposes. Some of that has been perverted into what passes as "private/public partnerships." The UDAG program, for those of you who are unfamiliar with it, is a program that amounts to giving money to build downtown Hyatt Hotels in major U.S. cities. That is considered a "public/private partnership" because the public gives the money and the private sector takes it. I find that a difficult partnership to accept.

I also would like something even more focused than a White House conference on privatization. I'd like to see a series of detailed, persuasive studies that delineate why and under what circumstances each privatization method works best. We have an array of different kinds of products to offer. We need to know which ones work best, why and how. This will strengthen our case. It will provide more facts to nurture the privatization process.

Also what is needed (and this is where organizations like the National Center for Policy Analysis, the Heritage Foundation, and others play a significant role) is a campaign to articulate and propagate the results of this research to the public. The way the academic sector comes in, of course, is in propagating the results over the long-term by reaching students. We are beginning to see people graduating from universities who view competition and privatization as important tools.

Next, and this was mentioned by Stuart Butler, there is antitrust. This is a powerful tool. I can see over the next several years an organized effort not only by the Federal Trade Commission but by organizations such as those represented here to challenge local governments—to identify instances where local governments are inhibiting freedom of competition by creating a monopoly for themselves and preventing others from entering the market.

Just as there was a Legal Aid Society, I advocate the creation of a Legal Raid Society that goes around the country raiding city governments for the purpose of injecting a dose of competition. I offer to any such organization, free of charge, New York City as a test bed to try out some of these ideas.

We ought to be picking targets. I think that at the local level transportation is a most promising target. It meets the criteria I have identified. It is an activity that almost every citizen has to do something about everyday, and therefore it is highly visible. Some of the more invisible city functions, like data processing, may be more difficult to privatize. But transportation, like waste collection, is a visible activity and a very promising target, because successful attempts to inject privatization ideas into public transportation will be visible and help promote a chain-reaction effect.

Social services are another good target, whether we use vouchers or voluntary action through "mediating structures." Social services lend themselves well to these techniques, and there is considerable interest in the private sector in applying them more aggressively.

With regard to education, I was intrigued by Madsen Pirie's comments about slipping into a voucher system. Given the anxieties in the United States about the performance of our public school system, we should capitalize on this concern to promote greater parental choice in education.

At the federal level, Peter Ferrara's proposal to create an IRA alternative to Social Security and the NCPA's proposal to create an IRA alternative to Medicare are the kinds of things that should be pursued. The constituency is already here, in the shape of bankers. Unemployment insurance through vouchers is another good target.

These are the opportunities. It is a matter of going out there and taking advantage of them, while recognizing we are in for a long haul. We have had some immediate successes and victories. But to really do the job it will take a lot of staying power and the creation and strengthening of the kinds of institutions that I see represented at this conference.

9

Opting Out of Social Security: Why It Works In Other Countries

John C. Goodman

I would like to begin by discussing two principal ways of thinking about entitlement programs that interfere with our ability to think about private alternatives. When free-market economists think about opting out of Social Security, they frequently come to the conclusion that it will not work. They think this for two reasons: The first is that they regard Social Security as a kind of chain letter—and they are quite right about that. It is a chain letter. It is also a Ponzi scheme. Our Social Security Trust Funds are, in fact, little more than accounting deceptions. For all practical purposes, every dollar that goes into Social Security is immediately spent—every hour of every day. No funds are being stashed away in bank vaults. For this reason, what we have amounts to a government-operated chain letter.

There also can be chain letters in the private sector, but private sector chain letters are short-lived. The thing unique about the chain letter run by the government is that the government has the power to tax. I can remember a decade or so ago, Paul Samuelson was writing about Social Security and came up with the brillant observation that Social Security is a Ponzi scheme that works! The reason it works, he said, is the government's power to tax. Now everyone is willing to admit that the private sector can provide pensions; it can provide pensions that work. But few of us would be willing to admit that the private sector can provide a chain letter that works. Only government can do that.

The second idea that interferes with our thinking about entitlement programs is that when free-market economists think about private alternatives to Social Security and Medicare they often come to the conclusion that private alternatives are in nobody's self-interest.

What happens when chain letters collapse in the private sector? And who are the losers? They are the last people who bought in. Who are the last people buying into Social Security? They are the current generation of workers. Workers of our generation are paying taxes into the system to support the retirement pensions of the elderly. Why should this group of workers say, "We will continue to support the elderly, but when it comes our turn, when we retire, we will not accept anything from the generation which follows." What this would mean is that the current generation would be required to pay twice—once for the current generation of retirees and once for their own retirement.

These two points are instructive because they can help us see our way out of all this. Let me return to the chain letter idea. When Social Security was started, it was not sold to the public by politicians who brought Paul Samuelson to Congress to testify that he suddenly discovered a way to make chain letters work! Instead, when Social Security was started there was a lot of hoopla about Social Security as a substitute for private pensions schemes. People were encouraged to think of Social Security as a substitute for a private pension. Even today, most people think this way. I have always thought: Why not encourage people to change their thinking and view private pensions as a substitute for Social Security? Why not do what Peter Ferrara is so good at doing—pointing out that if you pay into Social Security the return you get is very low, but if you have a private IRA and put money into it each year, eventually it will build up and you will be very well off.

Proponents of a private alternative are helped in this by a fundamental principle: In a mature Social Security system there is a theoretical limit to the rate of return each generation can earn on its investment. By a mature system I mean one in which there is net population growth and each generation essentially gets the same deal as every succeeding generation. In such a system, each generation gets a rate of return from their Social Security dollars equal to the current rate of increase in real wages. Historically, the rate of return on capital has been two, three or four times greater than the increase in wages. Being forced into a system with such a low rate of return, when the market is paying much higher, means each generation is losing. They are being forced into a system where they are worse off than had they put those same dollars into the private capital market.

At the beginning, when Social Security was in its early years, this was not the case. The first people who retired on Social Security made out like bandits. The first Social Security retiree was Ida Fuller, who paid $23 in Social Security taxes, and received nearly $250,000 in Social Security benefits. That is a good rate of return! For this generation of workers, however, the return is going to be much different. In present calculations, the rate of return is often negative, and these calculations often are based on very conservative assumptions. By this I mean that it is not unusual, in fact it is very common, for people to calculate the present value of Social Security using an interest rate equivalent to the interest rate being paid on government bonds. What this amounts to is the assumption that the government is as unlikely to default on Social Security as it is on a government bond. I do not think there is anyone who seriously thinks those two risks are equivalent. I think we all would admit the government is far more likely to default on Social Security. The assumptions being made in calculating Social Security's present worth are way too conservative. Polls taken of the young population show that they view the system as very risky—more risky, for example, than investments in private pensions. If we used a more realistic rate of interest to calculate the present value of Social Security, we would find that it is very negative for young workers.

What about the problem of this generation paying twice? Well, in the first place, generations do not make decisions as generations. That is an important point to remember when thinking about private alternatives to Social Security and Medicare. Even if we were to make a decision as a generation, it is not clear to me what kind of decision we might make. Many of you are familiar with the estimates produced by Haeworth Robertson, former Chief Actuary for the Social Security Administration, who calculated what payroll taxes will have to be in the next century. Robertson used three sets of assumptions routinely used by the Social Security Administration: pessimistic, optimistic, and intermediate. The pessimistic assumptions always turn out to be closer to the truth than the other two; in fact, the pessimistic assumptions frequently turn out to be optimistic compared to what actually exists. On the basis of the pessimistic assumptions, Robertson predicted that future payroll taxes may have to be between 40 and 50 percent of income to pay for the promises that we are making under Social Security and Medicare right now. These pessimistic assumptions, by the way, are not by any means the worst thing that can happen. They do not take into account the possibility of radical medical advances that would slow the aging process or cure cancer and other diseases. Of course for most of us, these possibilities are normally thought of as optimistic, but from the point of view of financing Social Security they are pessimistic.

It is also important to remember that 70 years from now, children entering the first grade today will be in retirement, so we are talking about the lives of real people.

In Great Britain and Chile, there are three principles that characterize the opting out schemes that currently exist.These are principles we must not overlook in considering our own private alternative. The first principle is that promised benefits must be paid. We are not going to succeed with opting out schemes that say to the elderly, "We are going to cut you off." Maybe we can cut back on benefits a little bit and maybe we can play with the indexing provisions, but not very much. Frankly, Peter Ferrara and I have always thought that it is suicidal to scare the elderly and make them nervous. Instead, a more effective approach in promoting privatization is to argue that it will secure the future of Social Security. That is what they did in Britain. British officials did not say it was going to destroy Social Security; they said it was a plan to make Social Security secure. They said, "The system is in trouble, and we are going to make it better." That must be the American approach as well. The political strategy is to assure the elderly that you are not going to take their benefits away from them; that you are going to make it more likely that those benefits will be paid.

The second principle is that the private alternative has got to be a choice that is voluntary, at least for everybody who already has paid taxes into Social Security. You cannot say, "We are going to throw you out of the system." You have to leave the option open to them. Maybe you can do what they did in Chile, each new generation of workers entering the labor market (people who have never paid any taxes into the system) automatically is in the private program.

The third principle is: If you are going to give people a choice, then you have to have a differential tax. You have to make it to their financial advantage to opt out of the system. Essentially you will be telling them, "If you want to be in the system, you are going to have to pay a high payroll tax, or a high income tax." The individual will calculate and discover that on the whole he is better off opting out of the system. In my study of the British Social Security System, I calculated the rate of return that workers earned at different age levels and different income levels. I did this to determine how well workers did outside of the system, as well as how they did inside the system. I showed it to a top official at the Department of Health and Human Services, who looked at it and was very irritated by the entire enterprise. He said, "We do not generally think it is a good idea to encourage workers to calculate what kind of rate of return they get in the system."

True enough. They don't. Nonetheless, in Britain, on the average there is a seven percent difference in payroll taxes; the differential is between participating in the state-run pension system and being out of the system. This economic incentive is crucial because that is what it took to make it to the advantage of most workers in Britain to opt out.

Because of the need to create a financial advantage to opting out, some people see a conflict between the goal of flat-rate tax and the goal of creating alternatives to Social Security and Medicare. I do not agree there has to be conflict. It is true that in most of the proposals made so far there is a conflict. Peter Ferrara's proposal to create a Super IRA alternative to Social Security is inconsistent with a flat-rate tax. The medical IRA (MIRA) alternative to Medicare proposal put forth by Peter Ferrara, Gerald Musgrave, Richard Rahn and myself also is inconsistent with a flat-tax rate. This is because we proposed to give people a tax credit of about $500 a year for opting out of Medicare. We chose to do this through the federal income tax system because the system already is in place. We already have monitoring devices and an efficient way to operate the program without creating a new bureaucracy.

However, we could have ignored the income tax system, proposed that anyone who opted out of Medicare would get an annual check from the government for deposit into their MIRA account, and have them go ahead and pay the income taxes they otherwise would have paid. Our

MIRA proposal would be just as effective had we gone this route. As such, this private alternative is not necessarily in conflict with the goal of a flat-rate tax.

For pension benefits, two potential role models for the U.S. are the opting out schemes in Great Britain and Chile. In Britain there are what is known as upper and lower Social Security tiers. The lower or basic tier is comparable to a minimum pension benefit. Everybody pays into it, and at retirement everybody gets the same pension. The upper tier is earnings related; the more you earn and the more you pay into the system, the more you get out at the time of retirement. Therefore, the second tier is more comparable to a private pension. It is the second tier that people are opting out of. The choice is not an individual choice; it is a company choice that employers make in consultation with their workers. The company agrees to provide the workers with a pension which pays benefits just as good or better than the benefits that would have been paid had those workers stayed in the government's system. Again, there is a payroll tax reduction, which initially was seven percentage points, for those who opt out.

There have been some minor criticisms, but essentially, as far as I can tell, most people are very happy with the British alternative. Pension managers are getting a good rate of return. There are even provisions for returning private pension funds back to the state, so that if you decide that you have made a mistake after having opted out, you can get back into the government-run schemes. However, most companies that have decided to opt out have remained out. The program consistently seems to work well.

Chile has a more radical plan. In Chile it is an individual choice, and there is a payroll tax differential which is even more substantial than in Britain. What Chile does is more like what we have talked about doing in the United States. Chilean workers can opt out completely by putting funds in the Chilean equivalent of an IRA. There are competing institutions which offer IRA accounts; workers put funds into these accounts and forego their right to draw government Social Security benefits during retirement. I believe that all new workers entering the labor market do not have a choice. They are required to be in the private sector scheme.

When I first looked at these two systems I came to the conclusion that the U.S. probably will have to do what Britain has done, because like Britain ours is a democracy and a developed country, whereas Chile is not a democracy and is underdeveloped. At one point I thought that we probably cannot do what Chile has done, but now I am not so sure. Maybe we can take the IRA approach, especially since so many Americans now have IRAs. As Ed Feulner pointed out, today more Americans have IRAs than the number of Americans drawing Social Security.

Because of the experiences of other countries, I am hopeful that a private alternative can become reality. What is needed now is an awareness on the part of public policy institutes in the United States that this is a realistic option, something we should push for.

There is one last point I want to make. We cannot do this by getting support only from country club Republicans. They are easy. It is important to realize that in Britain it was the Labour Party that passed the law which governs the private system. What's more, there was no opposition from any major trade union. The reason they supported it was because they saw that their members were going to gain. In the United States, Social Security or Medicare reforms will require the cooperation of both major parties and probably the support of all major interest groups.

One of the things we have done at the NCPA is publish reports stressing how minorities are adversely effected by these programs. You may be aware of our study on Social Security and blacks. In it we pointed out that when the retirement age is raised from 65 to 67, as Congress recently legislated, expected benefits for young black male workers are wiped out. We also calculated what blacks could expect from Medicare. Black males at birth have a life expectancy of about 64.8 years. They can expect to pay into Social Security and Medicare throughout their working lives. But on the average they die about two months before they become eligible to receive benefits. To them, the system is unfair.

But, if blacks are given a private alternative, and they calculate how they would do under it, they will find it a good deal. They can put money into their own IRA, and it remains theirs. When they die it becomes part of their estate. They become gainers under the new private alternative. The NCPA has had interesting feedback from the study; Jessie Jackson's Operation PUSH ordered lots of copies. They think we are a great institute, by the way, and doing good research. LULAC, an Hispanic group, also was excited about the study. They thought it was terrible what was happening to their members. We have got a major problem, however, in that what we are asking these groups to do is break with the old Roosevelt coalition. We are asking them to break with their traditional political allies, which is difficult. Nonetheless, you make inroads by showing them the facts, by saying, "Look, this is bad for your members."

We are hopeful that with more work and more communication, we can build a new coalition that will support the kinds of changes we have been talking about.

10

Social Security and Super IRAs: A Populist Proposal

Peter J. Ferrara

Social Security accounts for more than 50 percent of federal domestic outlays, and almost 30 percent of total federal spending. Adding in national defense and debt interest along with Social Security accounts for almost 70 percent of total federal spending. Clearly, the size and scope of the federal government will never be substantially reduced without addressing Social Security.

The huge amounts of federal spending on Social Security should be especially troubling, because of all Federal programs Social Security has the clearest, most widely utilized private sector alternatives—including pensions, IRAs, and life insurance. As Milton Friedman has argued, there is no reason why the chief functions of Social Security must be performed through the public sector. It is indeed a truly radical departure from a private, free-market economic system to require almost all Americans to rely on the government for the bulk of their income during a major portion of their lives—their retirement years.

Market-oriented policymakers also cannot ignore Social Security, because the program just will not let them. As discussed below, on its present course the program is likely to continue to fall into periodic financial crises in the future. Within the present policy framework, those favoring limited government will be forced repeatedly to resist inexorable payroll tax increases, with nothing to offer as an alternative but politically disastrous benefit cuts. This is playing the issue on the home field of the Liberal Welfare State. Imaginative leadership for the market must shift the issue to entirely different, more amenable ground, breaking out of the traditional tax increase/benefit cut dilemma.

The Need for Reform

Social Security itself remains plagued by overwhelming problems which demand fundamental reform. Indeed, while most public discussion has focused on the financing problems of the program, a new, possibly even more destabilizing problem has been developing. The rate of return paid by Social Security has been falling steadily. For those entering the work force today, even if all of Social Security's benefits are somehow paid, the program still will be a miserable deal. This is true even though today's retirees are still getting a good deal from the program.

The developing problem is a natural consequence of Social Security's "pay-as-you-go" method of operation, where the taxes paid into the program are not saved and invested to pay the future benefits of today's workers, but instead are paid out immediately to finance the benefits of current beneficiaries. The taxes of future generations of workers will be used to finance the benefits of today's workers.

We can trace from the beginning of Social Security how this method of operation has led to an inevitable collapse of returns. Workers retiring in the early years of the program had to pay Social Security taxes for only part of their working careers. Also, the tax burden in those years was quite low. The maximum annual Social Security tax, including both the employer and employee shares, was $189 as late as 1958, and $348 as late as 1965. But because the program is run on a pay-as-you-go basis, the benefits paid to these early retirees were not limited to what could be paid based on their own past taxes. These retirees instead were paid full benefits out of the taxes of those still working. Their benefits consequently represented a high return on the taxes they did pay.

Over time, however, this return naturally began to fall as workers began paying higher taxes and for longer periods of time during their working careers. For today's retirees, as noted, the program's benefits still represent an above-market return on the taxes that they and their employers paid into the system. But those entering the work force today must pay taxes of several thousand dollars a year for their entire working careers. Today the maximum annual tax, including employer and employee payments, is almost $5,600; it will be more than $8,000 by the end of the decade. For most of these young workers, the real rate of return promised by Social Security under current law is one percent. For two-earner couples or maximum-income workers—a large portion of the rising generation—

the promised real return is practically zero, or even negative in many cases.

If young workers entering the work force today could invest all of their Social Security tax money, including the employer's share, into IRAs and earn the returns historically received by broad-based stock market investments, most would receive three to six times the retirement benefits promised under Social Security. They also could at least match the other types of benefits provided by the program. Career minimum-wage earners would receive about twice the retirement benefits, while a maximum-income couple would receive at least eight times the benefits.

Moreover, it is still quite doubtful whether the already inadequate Social Security returns currently promised to today's young workers will ever be paid. The Social Security Administration's own most recent projections under the widely cited, "intermediate", Alternative IIB assumptions indicate that the entire combined program (including the Hospital Insurance portion of Social Security) would become unable to pay promised benefits by the year 2026, before those entering the work force today are retired. By 2035, Social Security expenditures would be running almost 50 percent greater than revenues each year. Over the entire 75-year projection period, the program as a whole would run a cumulative deficit 50 percent greater than the total amount raised in new revenue or by the cut in benefits over the same period by the 1983 Social Security rescue legislation. Paying all of the benefits promised to young workers entering the work force today would require that the total Social Security payroll tax rate (which includes both the employer and employee shares) be more than 23 percent, compared to 14.1 percent today.

Under the so-called "pessimistic" Alternative III assumptions, the entire combined Social Security program would be unable to pay full benefits by 1998. By 2035, when those entering the work force today will be in retirement, Social Security's annual expenditures would be running two and one-third times greater than revenues. The cumulative deficit over the 75-year projection period would be four and one-half times larger than the financial gap addressed by the 1983 legislation. In order to pay all of the benefits promised to people entering the work force today, under these projections the combined employer/employee Social Security payroll tax rate would have to be raised to 37.5 percent. This would mean a total Social Security annual tax, split between employer and employee, of $7,500 for a worker making $20,000.

Many observers believe that these Alternative III projections are in fact the most realistic. But at the very least, by publishing these projections the Federal government itself is officially admitting that the need for tax rates close to 40 percent to pay the benefits for today's young workers is certainly possible, for there would be no purpose in publishing impossible projections. And if such tax rates are at least possible, then we are all in big trouble. We should be making changes now to eliminate any practical possibility of the need for such tax rates.

In addition, the benefit structure of Social Security is grossly inequitable. Two workers paying the exact same taxes into Social Security over their working careers may receive widely different benefit amounts. As John Goodman has pointed out, blacks and other minorities with below-average life expectancies tend to receive lower returns from the program than the rest of the population. This is because blacks on average live fewer years in retirement and thus receive fewer benefits.

Social Security also seriously damages the economy, destroying jobs and economic growth. A primary agent of this destruction is the Social Security payroll tax. To the extent the tax is borne by employers, it discourages them from hiring. To the extent the tax is borne by employees, it discourages them from working. Either way, the result is less employment, and consequently less output. The payroll tax is nothing more than a tax on employment, and here as elsewhere the result of taxing something is that there is less of it.

As I mentioned earlier, the maximum annual payroll tax is almost $5,600, and scheduled to rise to almost $8,000 by the end of the decade. For at least half of all workers covered by Social Security, the total combined payroll tax is more than they pay in federal income tax. In 1983, payroll tax revenues, drawn primarily from low and moderate income workers, were over 70 percent greater than total Federal corporate and business tax revenues. In a society deeply concerned about employment opportunities, this incredible tax burden on labor is ludicrous. Yet, without fundamental reform, the future holds in store only further payroll tax increases.

How could a program with so many problems have been so popular throughout the years? In the early years of Social Security, most of the working population had begun paying taxes into the program, but there were few benefit obligations accrued. Consequently, the program ran large surpluses and appeared financially sound. Congress could routinely increase benefits without raising taxes because of these early surpluses. Retirees were receiving high returns on whatever small amount of taxes they had paid in their last few working years. Small wonder the program was so popular.

The future of Social Security, however, appears very different. The program now has accrued enormous benefit obligations to the entire retired generation, with virtually no funds saved in reserve to finance them. Instead of appearing eminently sound, the program now will face periodic financial crises. Instead of voting windfall benefit increases, Congress will find that it periodically must raise taxes just to pay for the benefits that already have been promised. Instead of receiving high, above-market returns from the program, workers will be offered low, below-market returns, and in many cases negative returns. As a result, as the program matures, it will become progressively less popular, creating an opportunity for real reform.

A Populist Proposal for Reform

The key to fundamental reform is to recognize that solving these problems, and the many other serious difficulties of Social Security, does not in any way require imposing sacrifices on the elderly. Quite to the contrary, appropriate reform would strengthen Social Security and assure today's elderly that they will receive their benefits, while providing a more secure and prosperous future retirement for today's young workers, as well as the opportunity to work in a healthier, rapidly growing economy.

The first step in any fundamental reform should be to provide each worker at the time he retires a U.S. government bond stating his contractual entitlement to the Social Security benefits that have been promised him. All those already retired at the time of the reform also would receive a bond. The bond would not change the amount of the retiree's promised benefits in any way. It simply would embody a contract with the government promising that the retiree will receive his monthly benefit amount each month for the rest of his life, plus cost-of-living increases, calculated under the law in effect at the time he retired (or when he received the bond for those already retired when the reform is first adopted).

Congress would statutorily express its intent that the retiree will have the same legal status in regard to his Social Security benefits, as promised by his Social Security bond, as a U.S. Treasury bondholder has in regard to the payment of interest and principal on a U.S. government bond. Similarly, under the proposed Social Security bonds, it would be unconstitutional for the government to cut the expected Social Security benefits of a worker once he or she is retired. Congress would retain the authority to reduce benefits that apply to new beneficiaries in the future.

From a conservative, limited-government perspective, this proposed bond does not give up much, considering the practical political realities. For those already retired, it is hard to imagine any but the most marginal benefit cuts ever being attainable. Even minimal cuts would entail great political costs. It would be far better to renounce such cuts altogether, thereby averting the fears of current retirees.

The second element of a fundamental reform package would be to allow workers an option to begin relying on an expanded, "Super IRA" in place of some of their Social Security benefits. This can be accomplished by allowing workers to contribute to the IRAs each year, on top of any other amounts they may contribute under current law, an additional amount up to some reasonable initial limit. Instead of the usual IRA income tax deduction for these contributions, however, workers would instead receive a 100 percent dollar-for-dollar income tax credit equal to the amount of their contributions. That is, their income taxes would be reduced by one dollar for each dollar they contributed to a Super IRA. Also, employers could match these contributions, receiving a full 100 percent income tax credit for the amount they contributed.

To the extent workers exercised this Super IRA option, they would then have their future Social Security retirement benefits reduced. For example, a worker who with his employer contributed each year an amount equal to 20 percent of his total Social Security taxes would have his retirement benefits reduced 20 percent. In retirement, of course, the accumulated funds in the Super IRAs would pay benefits which would more than make up for the foregone Social Security benefits, leaving workers with higher retirement benefits overall.

The Super IRA income tax credit is meant to be in effect a rebate of Social Security taxes to workers who choose to rely more on the private sector and less on Social Security. But since the credit is taken against income taxes, rather than payroll taxes, payroll tax revenues would continue to flow into Social Security in full to finance benefits for today's elderly.

The option could start off quite small, in order to avoid a substantial loss of income tax revenues. The revenue loss eventually would be offset completely by reduced Social Security expenditures, as retired workers came to rely more on Super IRAs and less on Social Security. Long before this point, however, the revenue loss would be eliminated on net due to new revenues generated from the increased investment activity brought on by the new IRAs. Moreover, from the beginning there would be increased savings through IRAs, which would offset any temporary increased borrowing by the government to cover the revenue loss.

This Super IRA option then could be expanded slowly over time. Workers and their employers could be allowed to contribute additional amounts to their Super IRAs for the purchase of life insurance, again receiving 100 percent income credits for their contributions. To the extent workers did so, those who died before 65 would rely on the private insurance rather than Social Security survivors' insurance. Workers and their employers also would be allowed to contribute additional amounts for the purchase of disability insurance, again receiving 100 percent income tax credits. To the extent workers did so, they would rely on this private insurance rather than Social Security disability insurance. Workers and their employers similarly could be allowed to make extra contributions to provide for retirement medical insurance, rather than relying on Medicare.

Ultimately, workers could have the complete freedom to choose how much to rely on Super IRAs and how much to rely on Social Security.

Benefits of the Reform

Consider the benefits of the reform, and its positive political features. First of all, Social Security benefits are guaranteed through the Social Security bonds, providing a meaningful improvement in the legal rights of Social Security beneficiaries. Moreover, Social Security itself would be substantially strengthened. This is because while the program's payroll tax revenues are maintained in full, the program's expenditures in the future would be reduced substantially, as workers relied more and more on Super IRAs rather than on Social Security. If the Super IRA option is expanded rapidly enough, all of the program's long-term financing problems could be eliminated, even under pessimistic assumptions. Indeed, with the Super IRA option eventually expanded to the maximum, Social Security expenditures likely would be reduced dramatically, allowing room for sharp reductions in payroll tax rates.

At all times, workers who wished to remain in the program would have the complete freedom to rely entirely on the strengthened Social Security system without change. There would not be any reductions in Social Security benefits of any kind for such workers, or today's elderly.

Those workers who did opt for the Super IRAs could expect much higher benefits, more so the younger the worker. The Super IRA benefits, moreover, would be completely equitable, with each worker receiving back in benefits what he paid in contributions, plus interest, on an actuarial basis. These benefits also would be financed on a fully-funded basis, which would secure them against the financial instability inherent in Social Security's unfunded, pay-as-you-go system.

Workers also would have much greater freedom of choice and control over their own incomes through the Super IRAs. Workers could tailor their own individual packages of investments and insurance coverage to suit their personal needs and preferences. They could choose their retirement age with complete freedom after age 59 1/2. The Super IRAs offer instantaneous vesting and maximum portability. Workers also could choose to leave some of their Super IRA funds to their heirs, which they cannot do with Social Security. The Super IRA option combined with Social Security is clearly an overall system far better suited to our rapidly changing, highly mobile, highly diverse, modern society than the 1930s-oriented Social Security system.

The reform also would have important benefits for the economy. National savings could be sharply increased through the funds paid into Super IRAs, with a fully expanded Super IRA option producing potentially hundreds of billions in increased savings each year. Such a savings increase would in turn produce new jobs and increased economic growth. Eventual payroll tax deductions also would stimulate job creation and economic growth.

In addition, the more workers across the whole economy are allowed to accumulate assets in the Super IRAs in lieu of Social Security, the more equal the national distribution of wealth would become. If all workers paid into Super IRAs rather than Social Security, the national concentration of wealth would be reduced by one-third. Yet, this would be achieved not by redistributing existing wealth, but by providing an opportunity for the creation of new wealth equally distributed. Through the private IRA investments, each worker would be developing a substantial ownership stake in America's business and industry. This would revolutionize political attitudes. Instead of retirees developing a psychology of dependence on big government, as with Social Security, they instead would tend to support private enterprise and free markets, as would average workers watching their stake in the private economy grow.

Finally, the reform would sharply reduce federal spending, as workers began relying more and more on Super IRAs rather than Social Security. With a complete option to rely on Super IRAs, federal spending could be reduced by more than one-fourth. No other single reform offers the potential for such a massive reduction in spending, not only without hurting anyone, but indeed probably making virtually everyone better off at the same time.

Political Prospects

The proposed Super IRAs offer allies of the market the opportunity to break out of the current tax increase/benefit cut dilemma, and shift the Social Security debate to entirely new ground. The reform does this by seeking to solve the problems of Social Security by offering workers a better deal in the private sector, without cutting the program's benefits or increasing the program's taxes. The cost of the reform is no more than a temporary net loss of income tax revenues, with new savings to offset any increase in government borrowing that result from the revenue loss.

Structured this way, the reform would not take anything away from anybody. It simply would increase the freedom and options of workers. It is distributing candy, not medicine. There is consequently no reason why it should be anything but wildly popular.

The proposed reform should appeal especially to young workers, serving to enhance a somewhat surprising trend of increased support among the young for the market. And the strongest appeal of all would be to the politically conscious, young, urban professionals, or "yuppies." These individuals receive especially low returns from Social Security because of their higher-than-average incomes. Many are single workers who should readily grasp the virtues of the private alternatives to Social Security.

There is no reason why the reform would not appeal to the elderly as well. The legal standing of Social Security promises to the elderly would be enhanced, and the program's financial ability to fulfill those promises would be strengthened. The elderly also would appreciate the new opportunities given to their children in the work force today.

The proposal naturally should appeal to business, particularly to the financial industry. Mutual funds, stockbrokers, insurance companies, banks, and savings and loan associations all stand to gain greatly. Labor should support the reform as well. Not only would workers benefit, but the unions could benefit institutionally as well. Unions could develop pension and investment systems in which workers could pool their IRA investments, providing a greater institutional stake and sense of allegiance for workers in their unions. As John Goodman has noted, labor unions in Great Britain favored a similar reform of that country's Social Security system for these same reasons. (Labor unions in the U.S. originally opposed Social Security early in the 1900s because they wanted to use union pension systems to develop greater worker loyalty to unions, and felt Social Security would limit the role of these pensions.)

The proposed reform fits exactly the strategic themes and approaches for privatization that other participants at this conference have outlined. I think it is a proposal that we can begin to implement now.

James T. Bennett
George Mason University

Becci Breining
National Center for Policy Analysis

Eric Brodin
Lundy Chair
Campbell University

Eamonn Butler
Adam Smith Institute

Stuart Butler
Heritage Foundation

Inga Carus
Carus Chemical Co.

Michael Caslin
Washington Legal Foundation

Edward H. Crane, III
Cato Institute

Ed Dolan
George Mason University

Don Eberly
Republican Study Committee

Peter Ferrara
Attorney

Edwin J. Feulner, Jr.
Heritage Foundation

Richard Fink
Council for a Competitive Economy

John Fund
Wall Street Journal

John Goodman
National Center for Policy Analysis

Timothy Hallivan
First Western Corp.

Charles Hobbs
Office of Policy Development

Robert Huberty
Heritage Foundation

Carolyn Johnson
National Center for Policy Analysis

Willa Johnson
Willa Johnson & Assoc.

Sam Kazman
Pacific Legal Foundation

Tom Langhorne
National Institute for Labor Relations

Mike Maloney
Clemson University

Steve Masty
Republican National Committee

Jim Meitus
Office of Management and Budget

Gerald Musgrave
Economics America

Jeff Noah
Office of Congressman Robert Garcia

Grover Nordquist
U. S. Chamber of Commerce

Wally Olsen
American Enterprise Institute

Bill Orzechowski
U. S. Chamber of Commerce

Mr. & Mrs. Daniel Peters
Cincinnati, Ohio

Mr. & Mrs. Lovett Peters
Boston, MA.

Madsen Pirie
Adam Smith Institute

Robert Poole, Jr.
Reason Foundation

Daniel Popeo
Washington Legal Foundation

Gabriel Roth
World Bank

E.S. Savas
Baruch College

Fred Smith
Competitive Enterprise Institute

John Sommer
National Science Foundation

David Steinberg
U. S. Council for an Open Economy

Gordon Tullock
Center for the Study of Public Choice

Bridgett Wagner
Heritage Foundation

Jane Work
National Association of Manufacturers

Martin Wooster
Harper's Magazine

Peter Young
Adam Smith Institute

PRIVATIZATION IN THE U.S.: CITIES AND COUNTIES[1]

The explosive growth of government is a world-wide phenomenon. So are the problems that accompany it. Nations around the globe are experiencing more and more demands on their treasuries and a limited supply of tax revenues to pay these services. Increasingly, countries are turning to privatization as a way of dealing with budget problems.

Privatization means the transfer of government activities and assets to the private sector. It can be accomplished by selling an activity, by leasing it to the private sector, or even by giving it away. Britain began a major program of privatizing numerous state-owned industries in 1979, under the new leadership of Margaret Thatcher. Other countries, including the European nations of Belgium, West Germany and France, are experimenting with the idea. Japan, Malaysia and Singapore have major privatization projects under way. There have even been privatization experiments in the People's Republic of China.

The most extensive use of privatization techniques in the U.S. is occurring among U.S. cities. Increasingly, municipal governments are beginning to contract with private companies to provide city services—everything from landscaping and vehicle maintenance to dog-catching and garbage collection. Why are cities turning to privatization? Privatization is often politically practical because it doesn't eliminate services; it transfers them to the private sector. And, it has proven to be an effective tool for reducing government expenditures.

*Adapted from NCPA Policy Report No. 116, June 1985. [1]Among the earliest works pointing out the potential benefits of privatization to city governments are Robert W. Poole, *Cutting Back City Hall* (New York: Universe Books, 1980); James T. Bennett and Manuel Johnson, *Better Government at Half the Price* (Ottawa, Illinois: Caroline House Publishers, 1981) and E.S. Savas, *Privatizing the Pubic Sector* (Chatham, New Jersey: Chatham Publishing House, 1982). A data bank on local privatization in the U.S. is maintained by the Local Government Center, Reason Foundation, Santa Barbara, California. The first book to explore the political theory behind privatization and examine successful techniques for achieving privatization through the political process is Madsen Pirie, *Dismantling the State: The Theory and Practice of Privatization* (Dallas, Texas: National Center for Policy Analysis, 1985).

City administrators for years have been using private contractors on an ad hoc basis. Now government contracting with private companies is becoming a regular approach. In cities across the U.S., officials who once thought of privatization as a possible alternative are now considering it a necessity. Consider the extent to which cities now contract with private, profit-making firms:[2]

- 35 percent of local governments contract out residential garbage collection; 44 percent contract out commercial garbage collection.

- 42 percent contract out the operation and maintenance of their bus systems.

- 80 percent contract out vehicle towing and storage.

- 35 percent contract out the operation of day-care facilities.

- 30 percent contract out the operation and management of hospitals.

Private, profit-making firms are now under contract with cities to manage cemetaries, museums, parks, tennis courts, swimming pools, and arts and cultural centers. Profit-making firms also are under contract to repair streets, control traffic, provide ambulance service, fight fires, provide crime patrol, manage public works, and even to manage entire city governments.

Table I provides a partial list of services now being provided to cities and counties by profit-making firms. What is most striking about the table is the length and diversity of services. Indeed, there is hardly a single city service that is not being contracted out to a private firm somewhere in the U.S.

The major reason why cities are privatizing their services is an economic one: to reduce the strain on tight budgets at a time when voters are

[2]Carl F. Valente and Lydia D. Manchester of Management Information Service, *Rethinking Local Services: Examining Alternative Delivery Approaches* (Washington, D.C.: International City Management Association, 1984) p.XV.

resisting higher taxes. City governments that are awash with cash rarely privatize anything. Two developments have spurred the trend: (1) growing demands on city budgets from interest groups which are becoming increasingly better organized and more skillful at exerting political pressure in pursuit of their interests, and (2) a cutback in subsidies by the federal government. As Washington scales back on aid provided to local governments, there is more pressure on city managers to find efficient ways of delivering city services.

The use of private firms to deliver goods and services previously provided by government has grown steadily in recent years. More cities are contracting out for the first time, and cities which already have tried privatization are increasing the number of privately delivered programs.

Table II shows the amazing growth in privatization between 1973 and 1982. In virtually every category of city service, privatization is on the upswing. In many cases, the growth rate in privatization has been explosive.

- Over the last decade, the use of private firms to manage parks has increased 2,700 percent.

- For managing recreational facilities there has been a 1,600 percent increase; for data processing a 3,600 percent increase.

It is worth noting that the numbers in Table II probably understate the growth of privatization, because fewer cities and counties were sampled in the 1982 survey than in the 1973 survey.

How far can privatization go?

- La Mirada, California (population 40,000), contracts out more than 60 city services, and has only 55 employees.

- The Trophy Club, a recently incorporated suburb of Dallas, has only one paid city employee—a secretary.

Yet by and large, most U.S. cities have not taken full advantage of the opportunities which privatization offers. As Table III shows, among major U.S. cities typically less than half of city services are delivered privately, and less than half of those are delivered by for-profit firms. Even when cities rely on private delivery, about half of the time privatization is only partial, with the city continuing to provide some of the service with city employees.

TABLE I

EXTENT OF PRIVATIZATION

Number of Cities and Counties Contracting With Profit-Making Firms, 1982

SERVICE	NUMBER
Public Works and Transportation	
Residential solid waste collection	482
Commercial solid waste collection	487
Solid waste disposal	342
Street repair	444
Street/parking-lot cleaning	133
Snow-blowing/sanding	180
Traffic signal installation/maintenance	408
Meter maintenance/collection	45
Tree trimming/planting	450
Cemetery administration/maintenance	77

SERVICE	NUMBER
Building inspection/code enforcement	111
Parking lot/garage operation	94
Bus system operation/maintenance	122
Paratransit system operation/ maintenance	129
Airport operation	127
Utility meter-reading	120
Utility billing	162
Street light/operation	501
Public Safety	
Crime prevention/patrol	50
Police and fire communications	17
Fire fighting/prevention	15
Emergency medical service	187
Ambulance service	304
Traffic control/parking enforcement	15
Vehicle towing/storage	1,028
Health and Human Services	
Sanitary inspection	9

SERVICE	NUMBER
Insect/rodent control	145
Animal control	89
Animal shelter operation	159
Day-care facility operation	153
Child welfare programs	28
Programs for the elderly	48
Operation/management of public housing for elderly	78
Operation/management of hospitals	108
Public health programs	58
Drug-alcohol treatment/programs	38
Mental Health/retardation programs/facilities	36
Parks and Recreation	
Recreation services	58
Operation/maintenance of recreation facilities	123
Parks landscaping/maintenance	162
Operation of convention center/auditorium	22
Operation of cultural arts programs	49
Operation of libraries	12

SERVICE	NUMBER
Operation of museums	20
Support Functions	
Buildings/ground maintenance	334
Building security	120
Fleet management/vehicle maintenance	526
Heavy equipment/emergency vehicles	483
All other vehicles	473
Data processing	337
Legal services	788
Payroll	172
Tax billing processing	137
Tax assessing	73
Delinquent tax collection	121
Secretarial services	66
Personnel services	83
Labor relations	348
Public relations/information	108

SOURCE: Carl Valente and Lydia Manchester, *Rethinking Local Services: Examining Alternative Delivery Services* (Washington, D.C.: International City Management Association, 1984), Table B, p.XV.

TABLE II

GROWTH OF PRIVATIZATION:

Cities And Counties Contracting With Profit-Making Firms

1973 AND 1982

SERVICE	1973[a]	1982[b]
Ambulance Service	169	303
Solid Waste Disposal	143	342
Refuse Collection	339	486
Hospitals	57	108
Street Repair	63	444
Utility Billing	104	161
Cemeteries	47	77
Data Processing (records maintenance)	9	337
Payroll	65	172
Legal Services	187	788
Public Relations	30	108
Recreational Facilities	7	123
Parks	5	142
Fire	2	15
Crime Patrol	2	50
Traffic Control	5	15
Museums	12	20
Number of Cities and Counties Sampled	2,375	1,780

Note: Columns are not exactly comparable because of differences in the sample base and, in some cases, differences in the definition of the service.

(a)Derived from Advisory Commission on Intergovernmental Relations, *The Challenge of Local Government Reorganization*, Vol.3, (Washington, D.C.: U.S. Government Printing Office, 1974) Appendix Table 3.A. Reprinted in E.S. Savas, *Privatizing the Public Sector* (Chatham House, 1982), Table 4.2, pp.63-64.

(b)Derived from Carl Valente and Lydia Manchester, *Rethinking Local Services: Examining Alternative Delivery Services* (Washington, D.C.: International City Management Association, 1984), Table B, p.XV.

TABLE III

PRIVATIZATION IN SELECTED CITIES

City	Number of Services Provided by For-Profit Firms	Number of Services Provided by Private Delivery: All Types*
Atlanta	10	24
Dallas	7	17
Detroit	6	14
Philadelphia	16	27
Phoenix	24	32
Pittsburgh	10	19

*In about 50 percent of these cases the service is partly provided by the local government and partly provided by an alternative means.

SOURCE: Local Government Center, Reason Foundation; Santa Barbara, California.

SEVEN METHODS OF PRIVATIZATION

There are seven major methods that cities and towns have used to privatize the delivery of services:

I. CONTRACTING

This is the most widely used approach. It most frequently is used for public works and transportation, health and human services, city support functions and some public safety services.

An important feature of contracting is that of all the seven privatization methods, it holds the most potential to reduce costs. The competition between firms bidding for a service contract drives the cost down. Another potential benefit of contracting is that it allows a local government to temporarily increase services, for example on a seasonal basis, without having to hire permanent employees. It also allows a government to use workers with highly specialized skills that may be unobtainable through its own civil service.

It is worth noting that a contract can have a negative price, i.e.a private producer can pay the government for the privilege of performing the service. In New York City, abandoned cars are picked up by private firms who pay the city for the right to perform the service.[3] The collection of waste-paper or other recyclable materials are other examples.

Many cities and counties contract with nonprofit organizations for certain services. According to a recent survey, at least 20 percent of local governments contract with nonprofit organizations for services such as operating day-care facilities, child welfare programs, programs for the elderly, hospital management, museums and other cultural programs.[4]

2. FRANCHISES

Under a franchise arrangement a government grants a private provider the authority to deliver a service within a geographic area. Users of the service pay the provider, not the government. However, the government can regulate the level of service, its quality, and sometimes its price.

Franchises are most frequently used for garbage collection and disposal, bus and airport operation, utility billing and meter reading, street light operation, vehicle towing and storage, ambulance service and emergency medical service. The primary benefit of franchising is that it allows a government to completely turn a service over to a private firm, while still allowing it to set service standards and rate structures. Because users of the service pay the provider directly, franchise arrangements work best

[3]E.S.Savas, *Privatizing the Public Sector* (Chatham, New Jersey: Chatham House Publishers, Inc., 1982), p.65-66.

[4]*Rethinking Local Services*, p.XV.

when there is competition among providers and when consumers can freely change providers.

3. SUBSIDIES

Many cities find that subsidizing a service provided by a private entity is a lot cheaper than when the service is provided by the city itself.[5]

- Garden Grove, California, saved about $72,000 a year by turning its cultural arts center over to a nonprofit group, to which some subsidy is given.

- The city also cut the cost of its youth counseling program in half by turning it over to a nonprofit organization.

4. VOUCHERS

Under a voucher system, consumers are issued a coupon with a monetary value that can be used to purchase a particular good or service. The food stamp program is a voucher system. Although used infrequently, vouchers have the potential for a widespread application.

A principal advantage is that consumers can shop with their voucher in the marketplace and take advantage of the benefits of competition.

- In Hennepin County, Minnesota, low-income residents can use city-funded vouchers at any licensed day-care center.[6]

- In Kinston, North Carolina, elderly and handicapped people can use vouchers to pay for cab fares.[7]

- Vermont has had an educational voucher system for decades.[8]

[5]*Rethinking Local Services*, pp.224-226 and pp.227-230.
[6]*Rethinking Local Services*, pp.231-235.
[7]*Rethinking Local Services*, pp.236-239.
[8]John McClaughry, "Who Says Vouchers Wouldn't Work?," *Reason*, January, 1984, pp.24-32.

5. VOLUNTEERS

As local governments face increasing pressures on their budgets, many city managers may be surprised to learn that there is a large pool of intelligent, able-bodied workers willing to work for free. Volunteerism is not a relic of the past. Nor is it confined to small cities. Many large cities are finding the volunteer efforts of teenagers, housewives and senior citizens can be used to save a lot of money.

- In Baltimore, deputized volunteers are used to enforce sanitation and building codes.[9]

- In New Orleans 3,000 volunteers are used city-wide in 85 different agencies.[10]

Virginia Beach, Virginia, (pop.263,000) seems to have taken the lead in showing how far volunteerism can go:[11]

- The Virginia Beach libraries use more than 100 volunteers, saving the city about $42,000 annually.

- Virginia Beach recreational programs are run with the help of about 3,000 volunteers.

- The Virginia Beach police department uses more than 60 volunteers in its non-uniformed divisions, and can draw on up to 90 additional volunteers trained to serve as uniformed officers.

6. SELF-HELP

Self-help is a variation of volunteerism whereby workers are the beneficiaries of their own efforts. Neighborhood watch groups are an example. Other programs often having at least an element of self-help include programs for the elderly, recreation services and cultural programs.

[9]*Rethinking Local Services*, pp.249-251.
[10]*Rethinking Local Services*, pp.252-255.
[11]*Rethinking Local Services*, pp.256-259, 260-262, and 266-270.

REGULATORY AND TAX INCENTIVES

These techniques are used by local governments to encourage the private sector to provide public services, thereby reducing demand on public revenues. This strategy involves reducing regulatory barriers to business, and reducing taxes or establishing new tax incentives for the private sector to deliver a public service. Although a frequent tool of the federal government, it is used infrequently at the local level. Applications include residential garbage collection, bus system operation, ambulance service and insect and rodent control.

PRIVATIZATION THROUGH THE MARKET[12]

There is an eighth way of encouraging private sector provision of goods and services. It often is an unintended consequence of government policy rather than the result of deliberate design. If government refuses to provide public schools, private schools will soon flourish. If government refuses to carry the mail, private mail carriers will do so. If government refuses to provide police protection, private protection companies will develop. We tend to forget that throughout the 19th Century, government was usually a latecomer in providing most public services—entering the market only after private entreprenuers had demonstrated that a demand for the service was there.

Today, market provision of public services is most common in areas where government provision becomes notoriously inadequate. Take police protection, for example. Since 1960, the number of serious crimes in the U.S.quadrupled, rising from 3.3 million crimes in 1960 to 13 million in 1982. The public response to a rapidly rising crime rate has been predictable. People have sought to purchase privately the protection and security that is not being provided publicly.

- In 1960, the number of publicly employed policemen outnumbered private security guards. Today there are twice as many private security guards as there are policemen.

[12]The statistics in this section are taken from Morgan Reynolds, *Crime by Choice* (Dallas, Texas: Fisher Institute, 1985) and conversations with the author.

- Households and businesses now are spending about $15 billion per year on private police protection—about the same amount that we spend on public police protection.

HOW EFFICIENT ARE CITY GOVERNMENTS?

Before examining the potential benefits of privatization, we can profit by taking a look at what city governments are doing right now.

Economist Barbara Stevens recently made an exhaustive study of eight major city services in 121 cities, in the Los Angeles Standard Consolidated Statistical Area.[13] One of the most interesting findings was that there exists huge variations in the cost of providing services among the cities—variations on an order that are virtually inconceivable in the private, profit-making sector of the economy.

For example, Stevens found:

- The cost of janitorial services in some cities is more than 700 percent greater than in other cities.

- The cost of street tree maintenance in some cities is almost 650 percent greater than in other cities.

- For traffic signal maintenance, asphalt overlay, turf maintenance, payroll preparation, refuse collection and street sweeping, the variations in cost range from 350 percent to almost 600 percent.

[13]Barbara J. Stevens, "Comparing Public and Private Sector Productive Efficiency: An Analysis of Eight Activities," *National Productivity Review*, Autumn, 1984, pp.395-406.

TABLE IV

VARIATION IN COST OF CITY SERVICES FOR 121 CITIES IN LOS ANGELES COUNTY

Service	Low-Cost City	High-Cost City	Difference In High And Low Cost
Street Sweeping cost per curb mile swept:	$ 6.24	$ 36.92	592%
Janitorial Service cost per 1,000 sq.ft.:	1.52	10.92	718%
Refuse Collection cost per ton collected:	12.48	43.62	350%
Payroll Preparation cost per check issued:	2.35	10.27	437%
Traffic Signal Maintenance cost per intersection:	843.00	2,801.00	332%
Asphalt Overlay cost per ton laid:	30.65	136.77	446%
Turf Maintenance cost per acre mowed:	39.02	193.46	496%
Street Tree Maintenance cost per trimming visit:	20.25	130.99	647%

SOURCE: Barbara J.Stevens, "Comparing Public and Private Sector Productive Efficiency: An Analysis of Eight Activities," *National Productivity Review*, Autumn, 1984, p.398

A natural question to ask is whether these differences in the cost of city services reflect differences in the quality of the services. As it turns out, Stevens found large differences ranging from "extremely high" quality to "extremely low." Yet these differences in quality were uncorrelated with amounts spent. In her own words, "Without exception, differences in service quality were not found to explain differences in service cost."[14]

What, then, does explain the wide variation in cost of services among the cities. Stevens found that most of the cost differences can be explained by the use of technology and management practices. She concludes that without any change in service, the average city in her study could cut its budget for these services in half. If the cities in and around Los Angeles County are at all representative of cities elsewhere, the implications of these findings for the nation as a whole are staggering.

Is there a way for city governments to set up procedures so that there is a systematic tendency to keep costs at a minimum? The answer is: Yes, by turning to privatization.

THE BENEFITS OF PRIVATIZATION

There is a wealth of evidence that privatization can save governments a lot of money. The fundamental reason centers around competition and business incentives to accomplish a task in the most efficient and effective way, thereby retaining the contract and profiting from it. These profit and loss incentives stand out in stark contrast to the incentives of a government bureau—a monopoly removed from the benefits of competition. Municipal officials have no profit-and-loss ledgers to guide their decision-making. Typically, they are rewarded according to the size of their agencies:the number of employees and the dollar amount of its budget. Their motives are centered around expanding their territory, rather than encouraging efficiency and reducing costs.

A second reason privatization can cut costs has to do with economies of scale. For small-to-medium sized cities, the area and population often is

[14] *Ibid.*, pp.399, 401.

not large enough to take advantage of economies of scale that large government-run services make possible. In these cases it makes sense to purchase the service from a supplier large enough to serve more than one city. On the other hand, for other types of services that same city may be too large to achieve maximum efficiency by using only one supplier. In these cases costs can be lowered if multiple suppliers do the job. Ironically, the one arrangement *least* likely to be most efficient is the one used by most cities: Services are provided by one supplier (city government) on the scale set by the size of the city.

The presence of multiple suppliers is central to both of the reasons why privatization saves money. Multiple suppliers mean competition. A monopoly that a government-provided service creates is largely insulated from consumer feedback (i.e. people's decisions on where to spend their money) and from producer cost-consciousness. Studies comparing the costs of public service show that the most important factor is not whether the service is delivered publicly or privately, but whether it is delivered by a monopoly or under competition with other providers.

Competition injects a whole new set of disciplines into a service that was previously provided solely by government. Simply having a contract go out to bid for the first time brings almost immediate changes. Local officials often find that the private supplier is far more responsive and careful about service quality than municipal workers who took it for granted that their department would be providing the service forever.

Garbage collection is one city service that has been studied on a systematic basis. A nationwide study by two Columbia University professors found that government-run solid waste collection was 68 percent more costly than private contracting in cities with populations above 50,000.[15] This study, together with other studies covering the U.S., Canada and Switzerland offer "overwhelming and clear" evidence that private, contracted-out collection is more efficient than municipal collection.[16]

[15]E.S. Savas and Barbara J. Stevens, *Evaluating the Organization of Service Delivery: Solid Waste Collection and Disposal*, (New York: Columbia University Graduate School of Business, 1977.)
[16]E.S. Savas, *Privatizing the Public Sector,* p.93.

For example,[17]

- A study of 131 Canadian municipalities found municipal collection was more than 50 percent more expensive per household than collection by private contractors.

- Private collection crews were found to be 95 percent more productive.

What is true for garbage collection also appears to hold for many other city services. Again, the most complete and comprehensive study to date is the study of cities in the Los Angeles area. After adjusting for differences in quality of services, level of service, scale of service, etc. Stevens found that:

- When cities do their own street cleaning, the cost is 43 percent higher than the cost for private contractors.

- The cost of city-provided janitorial services is 73 percent higher than when the service is provided by private contractors; for asphalt overlay, the cost is almost two times higher.

- Only in the area of payroll preparation do city governments keep their costs as low as private contractors.

[17]Terry Peters, "Privatization: Public Services and the Private Sector," (Austin, Texas: Texas Research League Analysis, Vol.5 No.8, August, 1984) p.5.

TABLE V

HOW MUCH CAN PRIVATE CONTRACTING SAVE ?
(based on 121 cities in the Los Angeles County area)

Service	Extra Cost As A Result Of City Provision *
Street Cleaning	43%
Janitorial Services	73%
Refuse Collection	42%
Payroll Preparation	-0-
Traffic Signal Maintenance	56%
Asphalt Overlay Construction	96%
Grass Maintenance	40%
Street Maintenance	37%

*These cost differences are adjusted for differences in the scale of service, quality of service and physical conditions under which the service is provided.

SOURCE: Barbara J.Stephens, "Comparing Public and Private Sector Productive Efficiency: An Analysis of Eight Activities," *National Productivity Review*, Autumn, 1984, p.401.

Although there was a significant reduction in the *cost* of the service, Stevens found no difference in the *quality* of the service when provided by a private contractor.

How did private contractors manage to keep costs down relative to the city governments? By using more capital, more intensive production methods, and more frequent incentive systems.Also by reducing absenteeism, giving supervisors more authority to hire and fire workers, and holding managers responsible for the maintenance of equipment, etc. In short, by doing many of the things that most business managers would do if they wanted to cut costs.

ALLAYING FEARS ABOUT PRIVATIZATION[18]

Some critics of privatization claim privatization will bring numerous damaging consequences, including higher costs, lost jobs and more corruption. Although it is always possible for a privatization program to be managed poorly, experience indicates that managed correctly, privatization produces good results. The following are a few principles that have been tried and tested in various cities with great success.

1. **Use of private firms should reduce costs.** Frequent and open competitive bidding on contracts will prevent private firms from gradually "padding in" additional costs over time. There are numerous examples of a contracted-out service being switched from one firm to another after a genuinely competitive bidding process. These include paramedic services, data processing, vehicle maintenance, and garbage collection.

2. **Privatization can help eliminate corruption.** The introduction of publicly advertised bidding on contracts (along with objective selection standards) helps eliminate corruption. Decisions that were once concealed from public view (particularly those made by city officials regarding public employee unions) are now out in the open and a matter of public record.

[18]This section is based on Robert W. Poole, "Objections to Privatization" in *Policy Review* (Washington, D.C.: The Heritage Foundation, Spring, 1983).

3. **Privatization can create jobs.** When jobs are eliminated in the public sector, resources are freed to create new jobs in the private sector. Frequently, the transfer increases overall productivity. For example, when cities use five full-time employees for a garbage collection crew when three could do the job, they are undermining the productive efforts of two people who could be producing something of value in the private sector. The transition to private suppliers may pose temporary employment problems. However, there are ways to alleviate these problems. One is to require the incoming private firm to give the displaced government workers first preference for the job openings created by the contract. The federal government's official policy on contracting out already requires this. When a data processing company won a seven-year contract in Orange County, California, it offered all employees a job. More than 98 accepted, although after two years staffing was down to 72 percent. How did the company do it? Not by firing, but by attrition and by transferring workers upward or laterally to other jobs in the company. The opening of new career paths was a key factor in keeping the workers' morale high.

4. **Privatization is politically practical.** Under threat from public employee unions, political leaders may shy away from privatization proposals. However, once the majority of voters see that a particular service is being delivered more efficiently at a lower cost (which smart politicians document and publicize) public support soon materializes. The current tax-revolt attitude of the public coupled with widespread suspicion of public employee unions already is working toward privatization's favor.

5. **Consumers are better served.** Efficiency, responsiveness and service innovation result from privatization. When public services are organized for profit, the benefits of competition (i.e. the threat of a loss of the contract) will accrue. If a new way of performing an old task will save the company money, the company will innovate. One good example is the case of Rural/Metro, the private firefighting company contracted by Scottsdale, Arizona. Rural/Metro pioneered a "portable pipeline" feeding two or three conventional lines from a portable hydrant. The change resulted in significant savings to the city because it could double the spacing between fire hydrants. Rural/Metro also invented a remote control robot for firefighting in dangerous situations.

CASE STUDIES IN PRIVATIZATION SUCCESS

Firefighting. The case of Scottsdale's experiment with private firefighting is one of the oldest and most widely-noted privatization success stories. Scottsdale has had private firefighting (provided by Rural/Metro, Inc.)since 1952. In the mid-1970s a detailed study compared Scottsdale with three other Arizona cities of comparable size. In terms of cost effectiveness, Scottsdale came out way ahead. Over the five-year period from 1971 to 1975, the average annual cost in Scottsdale was $6.48, or only 56 percent of the $11.58 per capita average cost of the other cities.[19]

In addition to Rural/Metro's equipment innovations, the company has made shrewd and brillant changes in the way it uses manpower. The company uses a mix of full-time and reserve firemen. The reservists are less intensively trained, are on call one week a month, and are called only for building fires.(Full-time firefighters handle the frequent grass and trash fires.) The reserve firemen are paid only for the time they spend training or responding. Thus, the company's manpower costs are much lower than the city-run fire departments of other cities, even though its wage levels are comparable.

Prisons. Pressed by the escalating costs of housing criminals, many states are turning to the private sector to construct and operate prisons. Nationwide there is a growing list of private firms getting into the correctional industry.

One of the first to enter the field was the Nashville-based Corrections Corporation of America. CCA runs two corrections centers—a community facility for juveniles in Memphis and a processing center for illegal aliens in Houston.

Buckingham Securities, Ltd.of Lewisburg, Pa., has received approval to proceed with the design, construction and operation of a 720-bed penitentiary outside of Pittsburgh. According to officials of the firm, Connecticut, Indiana, Kentucky, Maryland, New Jersey and West Virginia have expressed interest in contracting with the facility once it is finished.

[19]Poole, "Objections to Privatization."

Chief Justice Warren Burger recently called on prison officials to do what they can to transform the nations prisons into "factories with fences."[20] Here again, the private sector already is moving ahead on that front. "Free Venture" is the name of a number of projects launched in the late 1970s in which private firms contract with prison officials for goods or services produced by inmates.

Another unusual privatization experiment in the prison industry is happening in Minnesota. A private, nonprofit data processing company leases space in one of the state's correctional facilities. Inmates do computer programming for firms such as Data Control, 3M, and Honeywell, and can earn as much as $6 per hour.

Entrepreneurs of the private prison business say they can run prisons and jails more efficiently than public agencies. Many experts are cautiously backing the experiments. Said Anthony Travisono of the American Correctional Association, "Many public officials hate running jails and find it attractive to get the problem off their backs while saving tax money."[21]

Education. Sharply falling student scores over the last decade attest to the fact that public education is not doing the job. But while education quality has gone down, the budgets of schools continue to climb. An indicator of climbing budgets is the proliferation of nonteaching employees in schools. Some 40 percent of all public school employees have nothing to do with teaching—and in some districts that number is as high as 60 percent. Many private schools operate with less than 10 percent nonteaching personnel.[22]

In comparisons of public and private schools, the private institutions usually win out. For example, the city comptroller in New York compared the city's two approaches to educating handicapped children—in public schools and in private schools by contract. The per pupil costs were greater in public schools than in private schools—$6,196 and $4,730 respectively.[23]

[20] *U.S. News and World Report*, July 2, 1984, p.46.

[21] *Ibid*.p.45.

[22] Poole, *Cutting Back City Hall* (New York: Universe Books, 1980) p.179.

[23] E.S.Savas, *Privatizing the Public Sector*, p.102.

- According to a 1980 study, the cost of educating a student in a private school is consistently less expensive than educating a student in public schools.

- By contrast, the average cost of public schooling is $1,740 per pupil, according to the National Center for Educational Statistics.[24]

Private schools are succeeding where public schools fail for a number of reasons, all of which center around the quality of teachers and the students' incentive to learn. In public schools teachers are rewarded according to how many degrees they can accumulate, not how effectively they teach. As for student incentives to learn, declining academic standards have meant thousands of graduates each year cannot read, write, or compute adequately.

For years economists have contended that to improve schools and get equal educational opportunity, the government should issue vouchers that would allow individuals to attend the schools of their choice. Schools would end up competing to attract new students, and presumably would be judged on the quality of their education. Although it is not widely known, Vermont has had a type of voucher system for education for years. Today, 95 of Vermont's 246 towns have no public high school, nor do they belong to any of the state's 27 high school districts.[25]

City Management. If just about every municipal service can be contracted out, what about contracting out the management and administration of the city itself? The contracting out of city management is the newest and most innovative way to shrink government.

In what he describes as "private enterprise competition to bureacracy," a Florida entrepreneur has won contracts with two Florida municipalities to provide management, administration and even clerical services. Another entrepreneur in Florida also is winning city hall contracts to provide management and administrative services.[26]

[24]Poole, *Cutting Back City Hall*, p.184.
[25]McClaughry, "Who Says Vouchers Wouldn't Work?," p.24.
[26]Philip E.Fixler, Jr. "Contracting Out Management/Administration" in *Fiscal Watchdog* bulletin (Santa Barbara, California: Local Government Center, March 1984).

A third entrant into the field is the California-based Management Services Institute, headed by Douglas Ayres, a former city manager who pioneered the adaptation of private sector cost accounting to government accounting. The company already has completed extensive cost-accounting analysis for many California cities. Its staff is well-qualified. Employees include former city managers, financial directors, city clerks and municipal planners. The benefits of contracting out the management and administration of city governments are similar to the benefits of contracting out almost any other municipal function. They include reduced costs, more accountability, and better service quality. Private firms are able to spread the costs for the same management services among several municipalities. In addition, professional management firms can give more independent recommendations to municipal policymakers than a city manager whose job involves helping to meet the political needs of elected officials.

According to Ayres, injecting an entrepreneurial outlook among city hall bureaucrats usually requires a complete reorientation in thinking because "costs are an alien concept in local government." Nevertheless, the contracting out of city hall operations may become one of the most sought-after methods of cost-cutting through privatization. Reforms such as California's Proposition 4 require the strict accounting of municipal costs, which will necessitate the entry of management firms into this area. In the new climate of cost-consciousness among city bureaucrats, contracting-out may start to look more and more appealing.

THE REAGAN ADMINISTRATION'S PRIVATIZATION STRATEGY

The Reagan Administration's commitment to privatization is best known through its well-publicized attempt to sell Conrail, the federal freight railway. Less well-known, however, are the Administration's efforts to encourage privatization at the local level. For example, the federal government now spends about $870 million per year subsidizing mass transit. However, the Administration has been pressuring the recipients of this aid to look to private sector provision of services as a means of reducing costs.

In December, 1984, a regulation went into effect requiring local governments that get mass transit funds to allow private operators to bid for contracts to operate bus lines and other transit facilities. In addition, the Administration is considering proposing legislation that would require recipients of transit subsidies to turn over at least 20 percent of their operations to private enterprise.

So far, the Administration has made measurable progress on the transit front:[27]

- Private industry has taken over operation of as much as five percent of public mass transit—up from one percent in 1981.

- Nationwide, about 100 private companies now operate mass transit buses on fixed routes.

- Private concerns also operate about 400 van services.

- The cost of private operation averages from 35 to 50 percent less than the cost of public operation.

CONCLUSION

The growth of government can be halted and reversed by privatization. Dozens of U.S. cities already are experimenting with privatization (some on a large scale) as a means of improving city services and controlling their costs. Privatization is a solution for other reasons as well. It can create jobs. Consumers are better served. And it is politically practical.

The U.S. can look toward Britain as a privatization role model. In the last five years Prime Minister Margaret Thatcher has been "dismantling the state" on a massive scale, proving that even in countries which have strong socialist backgrounds privatization can work, and with support from the voters.

[27]Martin Tolchin, "Private Concerns Gaining Foothold in Public Transit," *New York Times*, April 29, 1985. pp.1,9.

MOVES

The Foolproof Formula for Creative Choreography

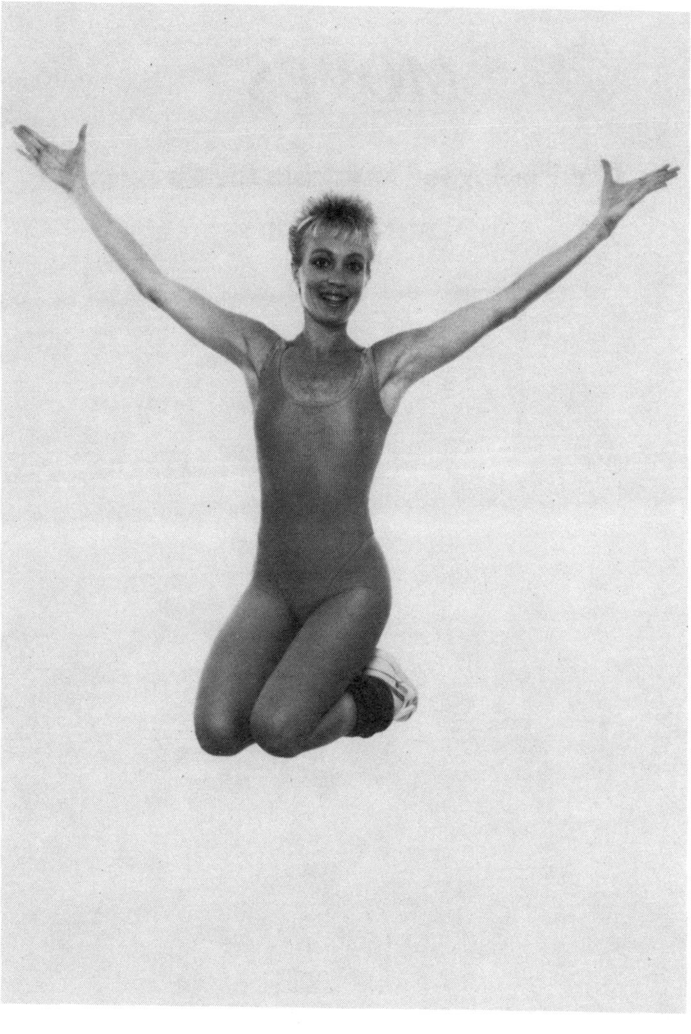

MOVES

The Foolproof Formula for Creative Choreography

By Candice Copeland

A ***POWER*** Book
CompuTh!nk Incorporated
Los Angeles, California

A *POWER* Book
Published by CompuTh!nk Incorporated
10394 Cheviot Drive
Los Angeles, CA 90064-4531

First printing 1987

ISBN 0-943559-06-5

DISCLAIMER: The recommendations and information contained in this book are appropriate for most of the population. However, the author recommends that any person embarking on any type of physical fitness program consult with their physician before doing so.

Design and Production: Jesse Berst
Cover Design: Share Reeves
Photography: George Monserrat
Models: Candice Copeland, Chet Vienne
Hair: Danal Ferris

Printed in the United States of America
by Spilman Printing Company
Sacramento, California

Acknowledgments

For their help on this book, many thanks to Neil Feineman, Jesse Berst, George Monserrat, Chet Vienne, Dan Ferris and Share Reeves.

For helping formulate my system over the years, thanks to the staff of Body Express, IDEA, AFAA, Merrily Smith, Joy Prouty, Linda Shelton and all my students.

Special thanks to Sherry Mandan, my friend and partner in developing Seminar Services and M.O.V.E.S.

And thanks to Mom and Dad for making it all possible.

To Douglas, my source of reference and inspiration.

Foreword

I first met Candice Copeland in 1984, shortly after she and the teachers she trained took the first Los Angeles City Sports Aerobics Expo by storm. As I covered the fitness scene for publications such as *Shape, Slimmer, Self, New Body, City Sports* and *The Los Angeles Times*, I heard rumors about the sophistication and exuberance emanating from this new studio. But nothing I had heard prepared me for the explosion of talent and spirit they displayed as they took both first and second place in the aerobic competition.

Two days later, I braved crosstown traffic and Melrose parking to experience Body Express firsthand. I remember the first class all too well. Despite my access to the city's best teachers, Candice immediately noticed that I had not been taught to keep my lower back on the floor during the abdominals. And my donkey kicks -- well, let's just say they made me look more like a less delicate part of a horse's anatomy.

That day, I thought Candice was simply the best educator I had seen in an aerobics studio. She reads, for one thing, and not just the popular and trade magazines but the medical journals and newsletters as well. And

she cares, and realizes that her best recommendation is a class that is fit, happy and injury-free.

When low-impact was just a whisper on the horizon, for instance, Candice had already filled several notebooks on the physiological and psychological implications of the shift to low-impact. Putting the theory to test, she had already scheduled a low-impact class, M.O.V.E.S., that she and Sherry Manden had developed.

M.O.V.E.S. went on to become the city's most popular and long-lived low-impact aerobics class. By the end of the first year, when most studios were getting complaints from their students that low-impact was boring, M.O.V.E.S. was turning students away.

This book explains why. Candice not only has a unique understanding of the basics of choreography, but has broken it down into a system that guarantees a physiological, individualized, constantly changing workout. As a result, rather than a series of repetitive routines performed on cruise control, the class becomes an exuberant celebration of movement and fitness.

Excitement, intelligence, unpredictability. These are the qualities that make Candice special. Now she shares the secrets of her trade with the information on these pages. As she does, she provides a framework by which you can constantly evaluate and improve your own efforts, as well as your peers. Which means aerobics has one more reason to give thanks for Candice Copeland.

Neil Feineman, Ph.D.
Los Angeles
September 1987

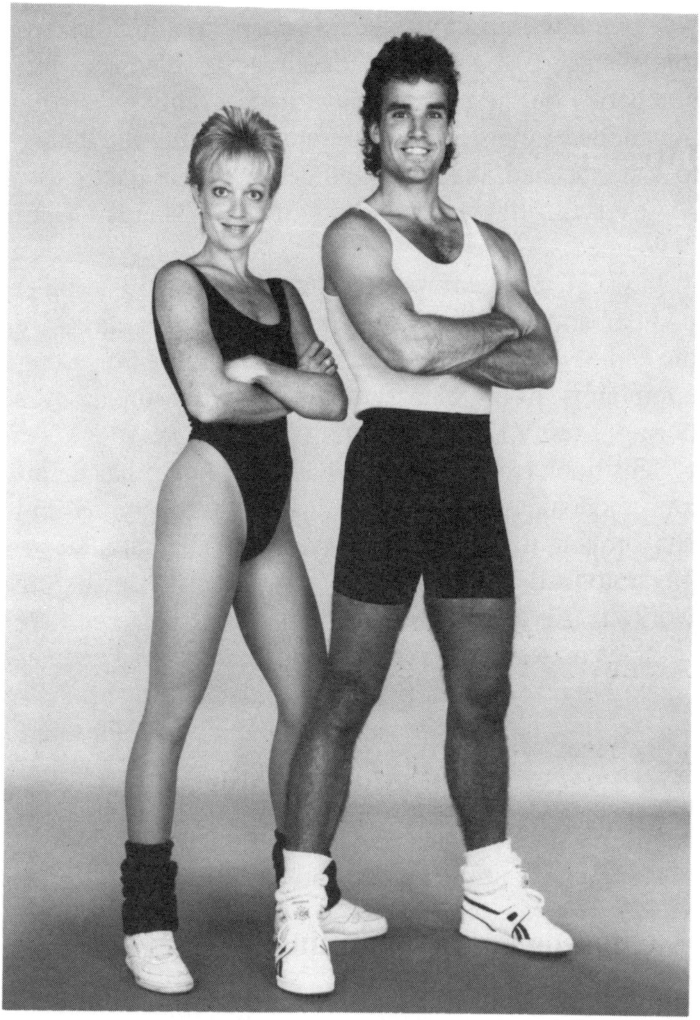

Table of Contents

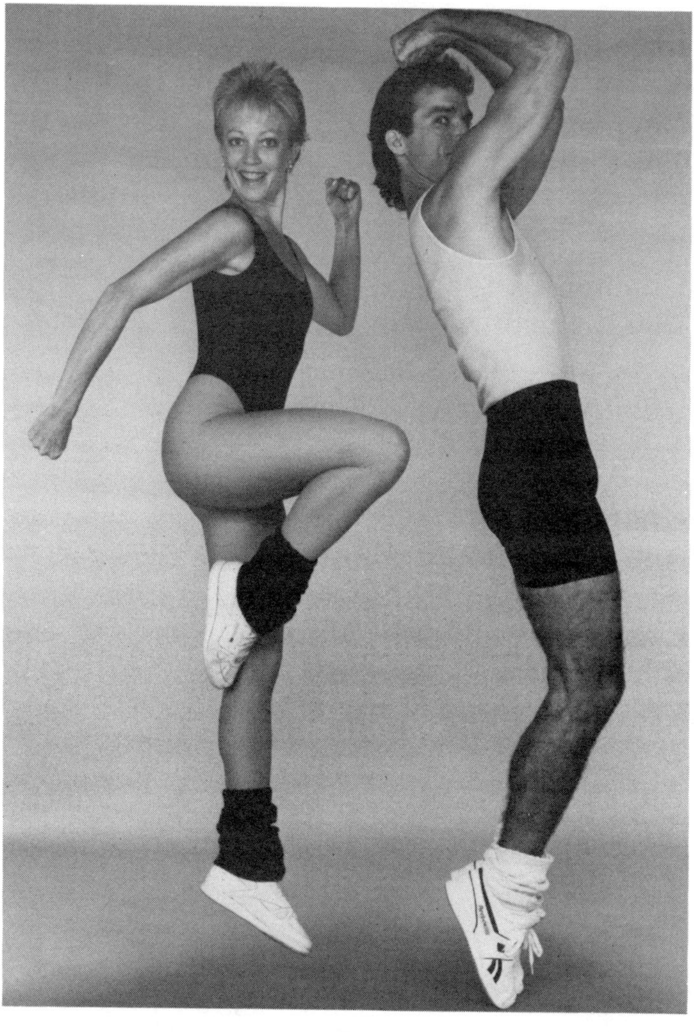

Introduction

What do you want out of your aerobic routines? If you are like most of us, your answer will probably include physiological effectiveness, safety and visual excitement.

Too many of us, unfortunately, do that by copying another teacher's routine. But mimicking another person's steps has several problems. First, everyone has a different style of movement, so what looks good on someone may not look or feel right on you. Second, since you are relying on a predetermined routine, it will soon get boring. And because the steps are already programmed, they may not fit the particular requirements or needs of the individual class.

By showing you how to break moves down into simple progressions, this book will change that. It will show you how to develop your own choreographic skill and ultimately your own style. This methodologyy can be used either for freestyle choreography or for pre-choreographed routines, as your needs dictate.

In addition to allowing you to have more fun in your classes, these skills will make you a better teacher. Whether you are teaching classes filled with seniors,

men, beginners or dancers, the process of breaking down the moves into the most elementary steps and then combining them into a pleasing and aerobically demanding sequence for the specific situation remains the same. Once you are able to do that, you can walk into any class and give the students exactly what they need.

If, for instance, I am teaching seniors, I might use big band music and simple dance steps. If the class is predominately men, I would eliminate the dancier steps and rely on more calisthenic- influenced dynamics. And if it was a dancier class, I would jazz those calisthenic steps up a bit. But in all of them, I would use the same basic moves and go through exactly the same mental processes to build the routines.

To do that, you will not have to memorize lists of steps and routines. You will instead learn the various elements within rhythmic aerobic movement. You will be able to break a complicated routine down to its simplest steps, and see how those steps can be reassembled into new variations and that can increase or decrease the intensity of the workout. As you do, you will be able to see the class as a whole and can vary the steps instinctively and in infinite numbers of combinations. By becoming your own innovator, you will become self-sufficient. And that will both make your students much happier and also give them results.

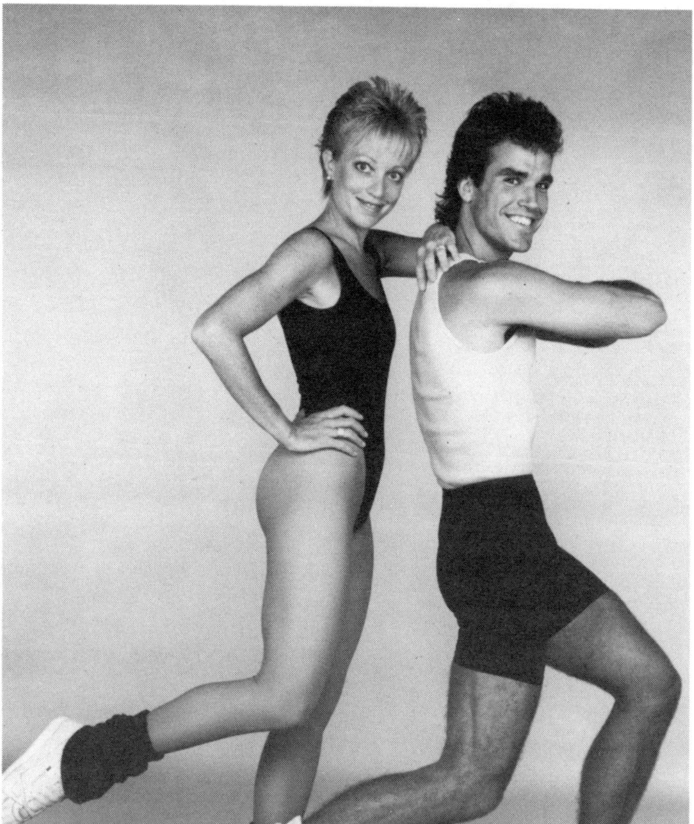

Chapter One

The Physiology Behind Aerobic Choreography

We all want interesting and entertaining choreography, but regardless of how exciting it is, it above all must deliver a safe and aerobic workout for each individual in the class.

Aerobic exercise can be defined as an activity which increases the body's demand for oxygen over an extended period of time, and produces energy at the same rate that it is used. As aerobic exercise becomes a regular part of someone's life, their body will gradually increase its ability to take in, deliver and utilize more oxygen, which in turn will help produce the energy needed to sustain the activity.

This oxygen is exchanged in the lungs, transported via the blood through the heart and to the working muscles by the vascular system. The entire transport/delivery system's effectiveness will increase with continued aerobic activity.

The energy needed for physical activity is produced by either using the aerobic or anaerobic energy pathways of the body. Which pathway the body uses is dependent on the intensity and duration of the activity. The intensity and the duration will also determine which available fuels the body will use to produce the energy.

These fuels are derived from the protein, carbohydrates and fats we ingest. These foods are broken down into amino acids, glucose and free fatty acids. Upon enterting various metabolic pathways, they provide the energy necessary for physical activity.

In long-duration, sub-maximal exercise, for instance, the aerobic energy pathway will be used, with fats being the preferred fuel for energy maintenance. We are able to work aerobically for sustained periods of time if the body is always able to meet its demand for oxygen.

In other words, the oxygen needed by the working muscle cells must be delivered and utilitized so we can continue the metabolic processes necessary to maintain the aerobic activity. The body then is able to keep energy production consistent with its immediate demands.

Energy needed = Energy produced.

The anaerobic energy pathway is used when the activity is short in duration and done at a maximal intensity level. Carbohydrates are the fuel source, and help provide the energy necessary for shorts bursts of high intensity activity. Because oxygen cannot be taken in and delivered fast enough to sustain this type of activity for an extended period of time, the body will have to slow down and rest in order to regenerate the energy so that it may continue the activity.

One of the by-products of anaerobic metabolism is lactic acid, which causes a burning sensation in the muscles and is a contributor to fatigue. Reducing the level of intensity or resting will allow the muscles to metabolize the lactic acid as oxygen becomes available and thus will facilitate the continuation of the activity at a lesser intensity.

Anaerobic training can be used for muscle strengthening and toning or, for example in interval training to raise the body's anaerobic threshold. The anaerobic threshold is the intensity at which the body is not able to produce energy at the same rate it is needed and lactic acid is built up.

Energy needed ≠ Energy Produced.

It does not provide cardiovascular conditioning or the metabolic training adaptations associated with aerobic training.

Our goal in aerobic exercise, then, is to allow each student to work at an intensity level that keeps the body working aerobically, thereby prioritizing cardiovascular conditioning and the burning of fat. When the student is working at this intensity level, we can say that they are working within their individual training ranges.

Training Adaptations

If you can keep your students working aerobically within their training range, they will notice the following changes:

1. Their **body composition** will improve. There will be a decrease in body fat and/or body weight and some increase in lean muscle mass.

2. Their **heart rate** will decrease. The resting heart rate (heart rate upon awakening) decreases as one becomes more fit. Similarly, the heart rate during aerobic exercise for a given amount of work will lower over time as that work session is repeated.

3. Their **stroke volume**, or the amount of blood pumped per stroke or beat, will increase. Maximal **cardiac output**, or the amount of blood pumped out of the heart per minute, can increase as the person becomes very fit. For a given workload (in which intensity and duration remain constant as the work session is repeated), the cardiac output will remain the same.

   The delivery of this set volume is determined by two variables: heart rate and stroke volume. The changes and adaptations of heart rate and stroke volume in response to training directly affect how the cardiac output "order" is fulfilled.

   The formula looks like this:

   Heart Rate (HR) X Stroke Volume (SV) = Cardiac Output (Q).

   When the heart rate decreases, the cardiac output can remain the same because there is a corresponding increase in stroke volume. This increased stroke volume means that the body can deliver more blood and oxygen with less beats of the heart. This increased efficiency translates into greater athletic potential, the potential for more total work and/or

more efficient work because there are less demands made on the cardiovascular system.

4. Their **VO2 Max**, which is the maximum amount of oxygen the body can process in a unit of time (usually measured in one minute units), will improve. When more oxygen can be delivered to and extracted from the working muscles, a greater amount of work can be done with the same amount of effort. Max VO2 is usually measured in millileters/kilogram of body weight, so that one's VO2 is measured relative to their body weight. This becomes a true reflection of their fitness levels.

5. **Blood pressure** may decrease both during periods of submaximal exertion and rest. The most important decrease is generally seen in the diastolic blood pressure, which measures and reflects the least amount of force exerted on the arterial wall at any given time.

6. **Temperature regulation** will improve. The body's heat transfer mechanism is more efficient and therefore enables greater exercise heat tolerance. The body can then cool itself more efficiently and endure longer periods of exercise at higher levels.

Not surprisingly, all of these benefits are interrelated. As the body adapts to exercise, it becomes an incredibly efficient machine. Since the effects are interrelated, improvements in one area are also reflected by simultaneous and related improvements in the other areas.

The Training Principles

This cluster of benefits can only be achieved by the implementation of a training routine that takes the following considerations into account:

1. **Frequency.** Three to five cardio-vascular workouts a week, each and every week, are necessary for maximizing the training benefits. Because consumers only repeatedly come back to something they like, the instructor must therefore make sure the class is sufficiently result oriented, safe and entertaining to make them return regularly.

   Note, however, that the importance here rests with the frequency of any aerobic activity, not just aerobic dance. The activities themselves are interchangeable. If, in fact, students can take three aerobics classes per week and supplement them with two swimming, biking, jogging or power walking sessions, they will not lose cardio-vascular conditioning.

2. **Duration.** The best strategy here is the principle of long, slow distance. Depending on a person's current state of conditioning, 15 to 30 minutes of aerobic activity can produce a training effect. Those who are more fit can extend the duration to achieve greater training adaptations. At no time, however, should the risk of injury or musculoskeletal stress outweigh the cardiovascular training benefits. People who want to extend the duration of their activities should vary the high stress or high- impact activities with lower stress or low/non-impact activities, thereby achiev-

ing maximal conditioning benefits and minimal injury risk.

3. **Intensity.** If the workout is not sufficiently demanding, it will not deliver the desired benefits. For conditioning effects, the activity should take place within the submaximal range, which is also called the training or target zone.

   This submaximal zone falls between 60 and 85 percent of the person's maximal heart rate, which is as fast or hard as the heart should beat. Our goal in class is to keep the student within that range, or at a steady state of exertion, for the duration of the activity. To make sure that happens, the heart rate should be monitored.

   To discover the submaximal range, we must first determine the maximal heart rate (MHR). Subtract your age from 220 to get this estimated number. Then multiply by 0.6 and 0.85 (60 and 85 percent) to get the target zone.

   Although this formula — .6 x (220 - age) and .85 x (220 - age) is widely used, there are other formulas, such as the Karvonen formula, that are equally, if not more, accurate. The Karvonen equation, for example, has you first subtract the resting heart rate (RHR, or the heart rate upon awakening) from the maximal heart rate. Multiply it by .6 and .85 and add the resting heart rate to that number. In mathematical symbolism, the Karvonen formula would thus look like this: .6(MHR -RHR) + RHR and .85(MHR-RHR) + RHR.

To arrive at these measurements, take the pulse either on the inner edge of the wrist at the radial artery, or on the side of the neck at the carotid artery. Count the number of beats for ten seconds and multiply by six to find out how many times the heart is beating per minute.

The pressure on the neck can cause some people's heart rate to slow down due to a reflexive response, so it is preferred to take the pulse on the wrist. Those who cannot find their pulse there may have better success locating it at their neck.

A less precise but adequate method of monitoring the intensity level is through "Perceived Exertion" tests such as the talk test. If the students can talk with only slightly more discomfort than in a non-exercise situation, they are probably in the target zone. If they can barely gasp for breath, they probably are in anaerobic metabolism and close to exhaustion. As a general guideline, working at a level slightly harder than what is comfortable places someone well within their target zone.

Keep in mind that these are general guidelines that are not necessarily suited for certain individuals in high- risk categories, or even for those people who have been inactive for a period of time.

4. **Specificity**. Aerobic exercise concentrates specifically on working the body aerobically by using large muscle groups in a rhythmic activity that can be sustained for a long period of time. Despite claims from certain "get-fit-quick experts," strength training,

which is anaerobic, cannot be done simultaneously with cardio-vascular conditioning.

Using light weights with low impact moves, for instance, is not done to build arm muscles but to place additional demands on the cardio-vascular system. Endurance and arm strength may increase somewhat, but the focus should be on pushing and strengthening the heart muscle, not the arms. If you want to build bigger arms, do it later, through systematic anaerobic weight training.

5. **Positive overload**. Your body gradually adapts to exercise. As it does, what was once difficult becomes easy and ultimately insufficiently challenging. To keep your workouts effective, you must increase the workload slightly so that the body remains challenged. This overload can be achieved by increasing the intensity, frequency and/or duration of the current exercise level.

6. **Reversibility.** The body cannot store fitness. If you stop exercising or exercise inconsistently, you will not see steady progress or any of the positive training adaptations. Consistency thus becomes the key to fitness. Working out six times one week and once the next provides fewer of the benefits than working out three to five times each week.

Injury Prevention

There are two basic types of injuries that happen in an aerobics class: those acute injuries such as ankle sprains that happen in an instant and those chronic overuse injuries such as stress fractures and shin splints that are related to accumulative, repetitive trauma.

The acute injuries frequently happen because of an accident. Chronic injuries, on the other hand, occur over time and can be traced to improper technique, surfaces or equipment or overuse. Treatment generally involves the RICE formula (rest, ice, compression and elevation). Since these injuries take time to heal, however, the best treatment of all is prevention.

Since overuse is one of the principal causes of these chronic conditions, it is a good idea not to either take or teach more than eight to ten classes a week. Variety is also a great strategy — having a few aerobic alternatives will allow you to get the maximal cardio-vascular benefits but diffuse the amount of stress the particular joint receives.

Wearing the proper shoes and working on proper surfaces (not carpet over concrete) will also help. So will the use of proper body mechanics, technique and alignment. The question of form is particularly important, especially on moves that are potentially stressful. These include hopping too many times (more than four, for most people) on one foot; any move when both feet leave the ground and land at the same time (such as jumping jacks); moving forward, back or laterally with a movement that doesn't naturally move in that direction (such as jumping jacks moving forward); straight

leg high kicks (that can cause arched backs or muscle pulls from kicks that are too high); excessive lateral movement especially early on the aerobic portion of the class; any position that causes the knee to twist and torque (especially potentially at risk with low-impact movement); and any type of movement in which the body moves in an uncontrolled or jerky fashion.

Remember that some of these moves are only potentially stressful when overused. When they are integrated into a well-designed, varied class and executed with the proper form, almost anyone can follow the routine without losing any of the physiological benefits of the class or incurring an additional risk of injury.

When the physiological principles are observed and are combined with the components of choreography we are about to talk about, they will provide you a class that is not only safe and effective but fun as well.

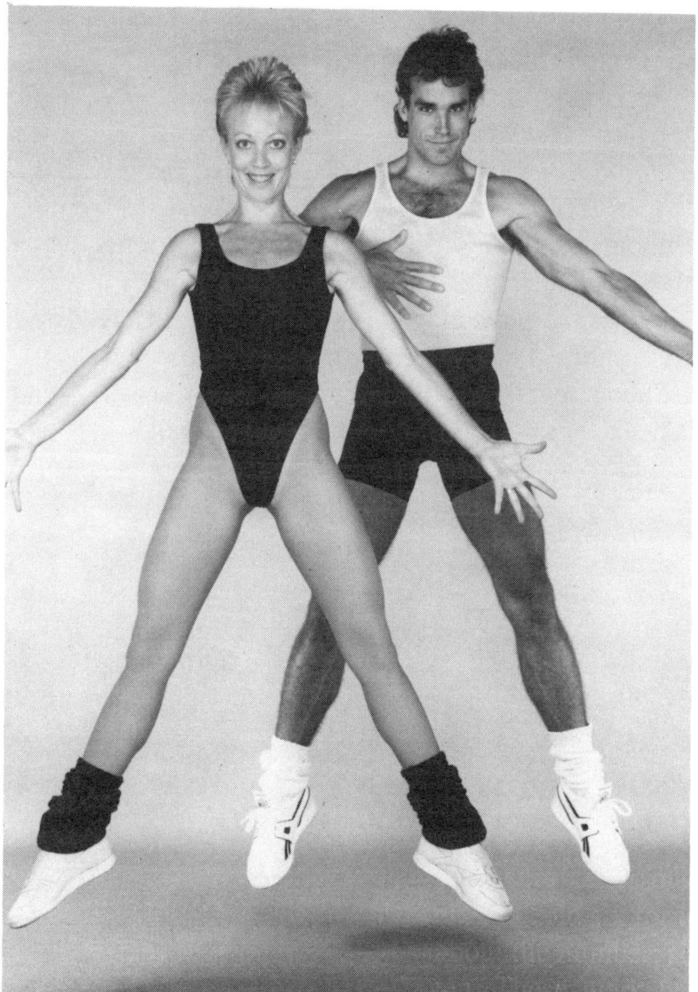

Chapter Two

The Elements of Variation

With this basic physiology in mind, you are ready to learn how to break down movement to its lowest common denominator. The concept is just like the lowest common denominator you studied in math class, because it is the simplest form of the movement. You break down the routine into these base moves so that you can see each component independently. Once each is isolated and stands out in its own right, you can then develop a base from which to start or return to.

The Base Moves

I use a series of eight base moves for high-impact classes, and six for low-impact. There is nothing magic about the number; some people use four, and others use ten. These work best for me, however, because they

give me enough options to avoid repitition but not so many possibilities as to become overwhelming.

For the high-impact class, the eight base moves I use are:

- Running
- Hopping (on one foot)
- Jumping
- Jumping Jacks
- Skipping
- Knee Lifting
- Leg Swings (Pendulums)
- Twisting

The low impact base moves are:

- Step Touch
- Push Touch
- Low Kick
- Knee Lift
- Walking
- Twisting

Everything I do starts from these base moves. Then, to put them together, I rely on five different elements of variation: lever, planal, directional, rhythmic and intensity variation. Along with the lowest common denominator moves, they should come together seamlessly in a class. But before that can be done, they too have to broken down into their component parts.

Lever Variation

There are two types of lever movement, long and short levers. Long levers work from the shoulder or the hip joint, such as jumping jacks when the arms are moving from the shoulder. These movements usually involve the full range of motion and therefore generally increase the intensity level. (See Figure 2.1).

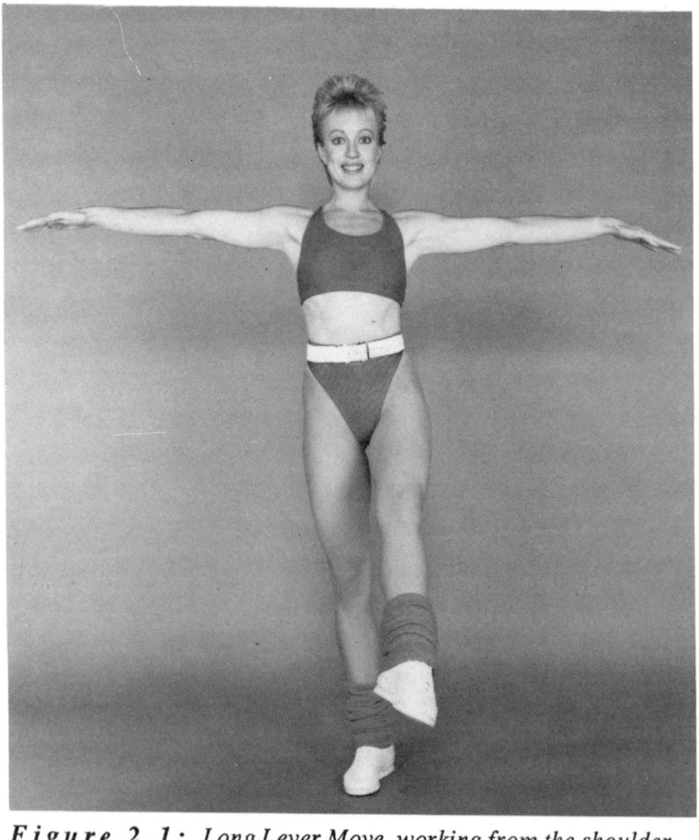

Figure 2.1: *Long Lever Move, working from the shoulder or the hip joint.*

Short levers usually require flexion at the elbows and knees. This type of movement generally lowers the intensity level because of the more restricted range of motion. (See Figure 2.2).

Good choreography uses both types of levers not just to balance the intensity and range of motion in a class, but to prevent injury and joint stress. As with any movement, a long lever motion such as a straight leg kick, is

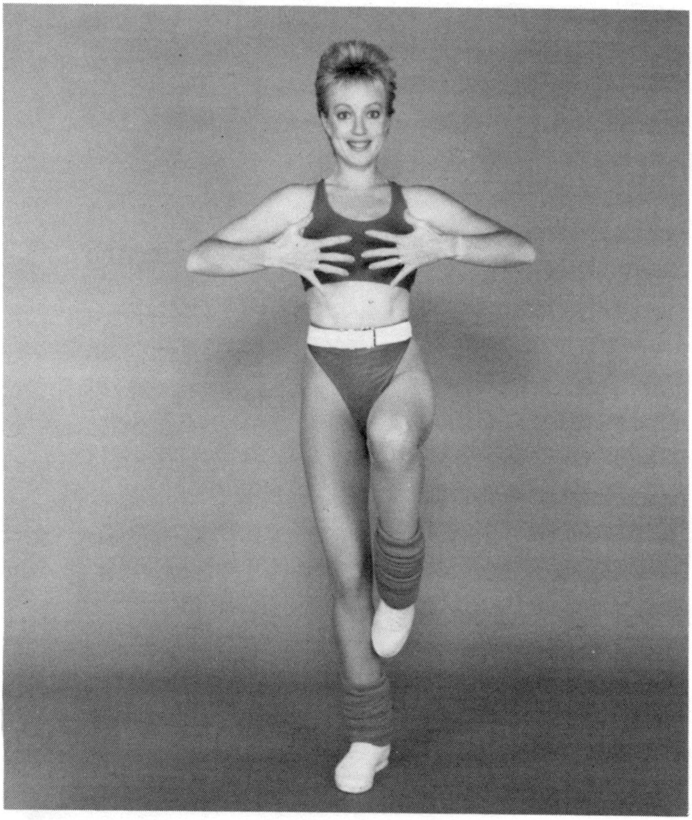

Figure 2.2: *Short Lever Move, restricting the range of motion by bending the elbows or knees*

not necessarily bad. When overused, however, it can result in injuries, especially since long lever movements can become momentum oriented and potentially stressful to the joints. Combining the two levers lowers the risk of this problem.

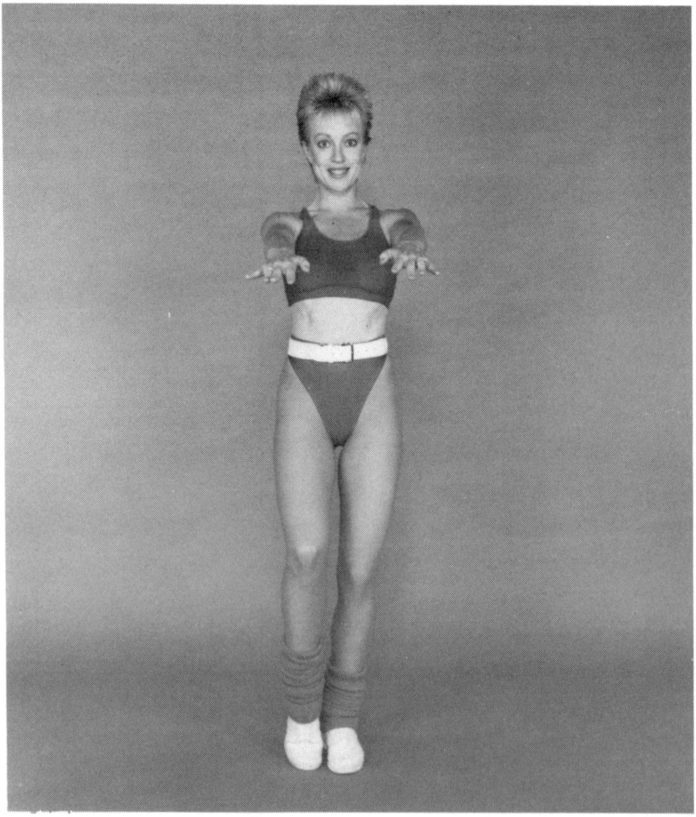

Figure 2.3: *Horizontal Planes, working side to side around the body.*

Planal Variation

The three basic planes at your disposal are horizontal (Figure 2.3), vertical (Figure 2.4) and diagonal (Figure 2.5). To help picture them, think of yourself enclosed in a plastic bubble. How many surfaces (planes) can you touch?

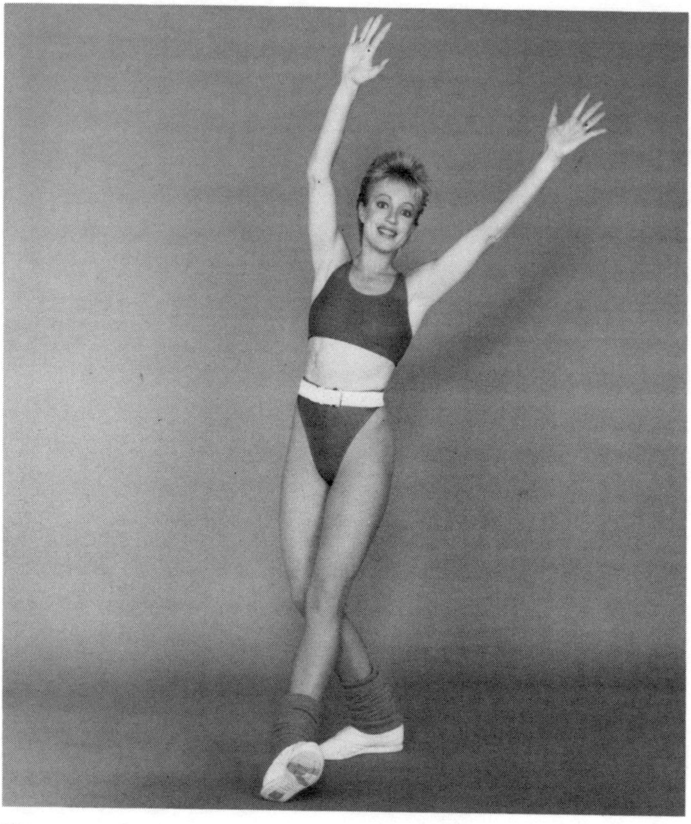

Figure 2.4: *Vertical Planes, working up and down or over the head.*

As you can imagine, there are unlimited possibilities for variation. Assume for a minute you are working in a vertical plane, with the arms over the head. One way to vary the plane is by moving the arms in front of you, or down, or side to side in high or low directions.

Planal variation is an excellent way to affect the intensity level without changing the basic movement. Just by moving the arms from overhead to chest level, for

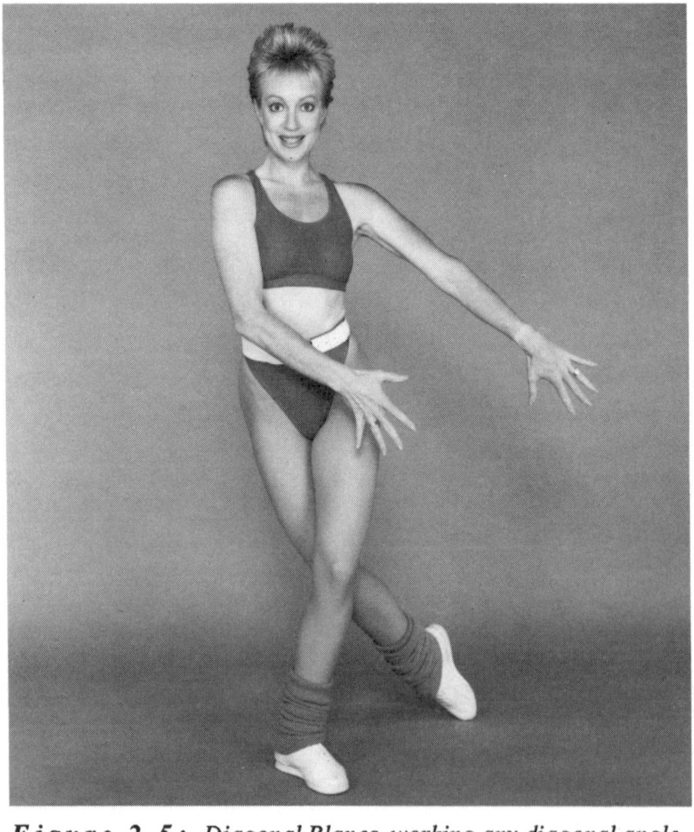

Figure 2.5: *Diagonal Planes, working any diagonal angle away from the center of the body.*

example, you can drop the heartrate a few beats per minute. This fine tuning of the intensity without changing the movement pattern keeps the class involved without confusing or disrupting them.

By combining high intensity planes (generally overhead;) with lower intensity planes (generally below the waist), a good choreographer can effortlessly keep the class in a steady state. By not staying too long in the higher planes, the class does not become anaerobic; and by not remaining too long in the lower planes, the class does not drop below a training rate.

When used well, the planes can thus keep the intensity levels within relatively small and effective fluctuations rather than big waves with energy-inefficient peaks and valleys. This becomes critical, because no matter how creative your routines are, they have to be within the aerobic training range or there is no workout.

Directional Variation

Directional variation works by simply changing the direction in which the body is moving. This is achieved by facing a directional point, or by traveling forward, backwards or away from an external directional point.

This change in direction varies the intensity level and adds visual excitement to the class. It is also a particularly easy type of variation, since the basic move is not changed, just moved forward, backwards or side to side.

Keep in mind that certain moves naturally move better in one direction. If you try and force the students

into a less comfortable position, you might add unnecessary amounts of stress. Jumping jacks, for example, travel backwards well, but are less suitable for forward motion. It not only is harder to take off with two feet jumping forward, but you can also jam the feet, knees or spine in doing so. As you practice directional variation, you will be able to see which moves travel best in the what direction, and then learn how to use them properly.

Rhythmic Variation

Rhythmic variation is how much or how little movement you have within a phrase of music. If you are marching to an eight-count phrase, for example, you can clap on every beat, every other beat, every fourth beat, at the end, twice per beat, etc. Each would sound and look different.

There are three basic ways to vary the rhythm: with sound, look and feel. If you want to vary it with sound, make a noise, be it a stomp, a clap, or a snap. Then see if you can syncopate the sound, or if you can accent the up or downbeat of the music. Any of these changes will noticeably vary the entire sequence of movement.

To change the look, you might try multiple reps, such as two, four or eight repititions on one side and then on the other. Or try combining multiple reps with single reps. Again, there are unlimited possibilities, especially if you think in terms of both putting moves in and taking them out. This tension between movement and the absence of movement creates rhythm.

The feel of the rhythm generally is either smooth and legato or crisp and staccato. A pendulum leg swing from side to side is smooth, for instance, while jogging in place is staccato. You can vary the rhythm by combining eight jogs in place with four pendulum leg swings, or with some other type of smooth movement.

Rhythmic variation sounds more complicated than it is, which is probably why it is so often overlooked. It is, however, one of my favorite variation strategies, because it gives the class the impression that they have been given a completely different move when in fact you have made only a minor adjustment. And because it is only an adjustment, it keeps their interest and at the same time makes them feel comfortable since it is still familiar.

Rhythm can be one of the keys to long-life choreography, because it lets you keep things simple enough that the class does not spend their time fighting complexity. Overly complex routines are not just emotionally frustrating, but also tend to drop the heartrate. By keeping the movement simple enough to keep your students working but different enough to keep them interested, you will be able to keep them coming back day after day.

Intensity Variation

Intensity can be adjusted either physiologically or psychologically. Physiological intensity, which is concerned with the body's physical effort, can be adjusted by using any of the other elements of variation.

Generally speaking, long levers, overhead planes, directional movement, and increased amounts of rhythmic movement result in higher intensity than short levers, planes below the waist, stationary movement and smaller amounts of rhythmic movement.

Remember that the bottom line of aerobic choreography is the attainment of a physiological steady state. This, not visual creativity, should be the basis for choosing the element of variation. Since the class is a workout before it is anything else, physiology considerations must always come first.

Psychological intensity generally involves the complexity of the movement. Complexity usually decreases the intensity of the work, because confusion and/or concentration typically decreases the range of motion. Make sure, therefore, that the complexity level is appropriate to the level of the clientele.

Whether it is a multi-level class or one already grouped by ability, the goal is to challenge but not thwart the class. The best way to do that is to gear the complexity to the middle or most intermediate level of the class. When in doubt, err on the side of simplicity, not complexity.

Even the most advanced students do not necessarily need additional complexity to challenge them. Ultimately they are more interested in physiological variations that result in a better workout. If it is too complex, they not only stop having fun but lose some of the edge from the workout.

So as not to lose them, it is better, then, to challenge each student by giving them specific instructions that meets their individual needs. Without changing the

basic move, show how the less advanced student can pull it down and reduce the level of effort and how the more advanced one can intensify it with resistance, range of motion and precision. This will keep them mentally alert at the same time it enhances the physiological benefits of the workout.

One tool I do not recommend you use to vary the intensity level is your own energy output. You don't need to perform; they do. Don't rely on loud music, forced hysterics or solicited verbal responses as a gauge of successful energy. Instead communicate what you need, and what they have to do. It is all right if every class does not have an emotional wallop, as long as every class is a good workout. If it is, they will continue to come back because you will be giving them something they cannot get anywhere else in their lives.

Drills

Drill #1 — The Exploration Drill

Take one basic move and one element of variation at a time and see how many moves you can up with. Pick any of the base moves, and set simple arms to it. See if you can vary the lever from long to short, or how many times you can vary the plane, the direction or the rhythm. Once you exhaust the possibilities of one basic move, choose another and repeat the whole drill. As you practice this, you should find that there are almost unlimited numbers of variations for each base move.

Drill #2 — The Rhythm Drill

To discover how much mileage you can get out of one move simply by playing with the rhythm, pick one of the basic moves and develop three rhythmic variations to it. Say you pick the step- touch. An example of one variation would be a clap on the touch. Another variation would be double reps or two step touches on each side with the clap. A third could be two step touches on each side with a single clap after the first and a double clap after the second.

Drill #3 — The Variation Drill

Perhaps the best single drill of all, this is most effective when done with a partner. Agree on one move and then have your partner tell you to vary the move, specifying what element to modify. Make sure that you change ONLY that element.

If, for example, you are doing traditional jumping jacks with arms over the head and your partner tells you to change levers, all you have to do is bend the elbows. It would be hard to do more without changing the plane.

This drill kicks you out of old habits and teaches you how not only how to build combinations, but also how to make one variation at a time. This is important because it gives the students a continual sense of anticipation without your giving up all your moves in the first ten minutes of class. Since that single variation changes the student's entire perception of the move, it eliminates repetition and allows you to spend the entire class developing new sequences throughout.

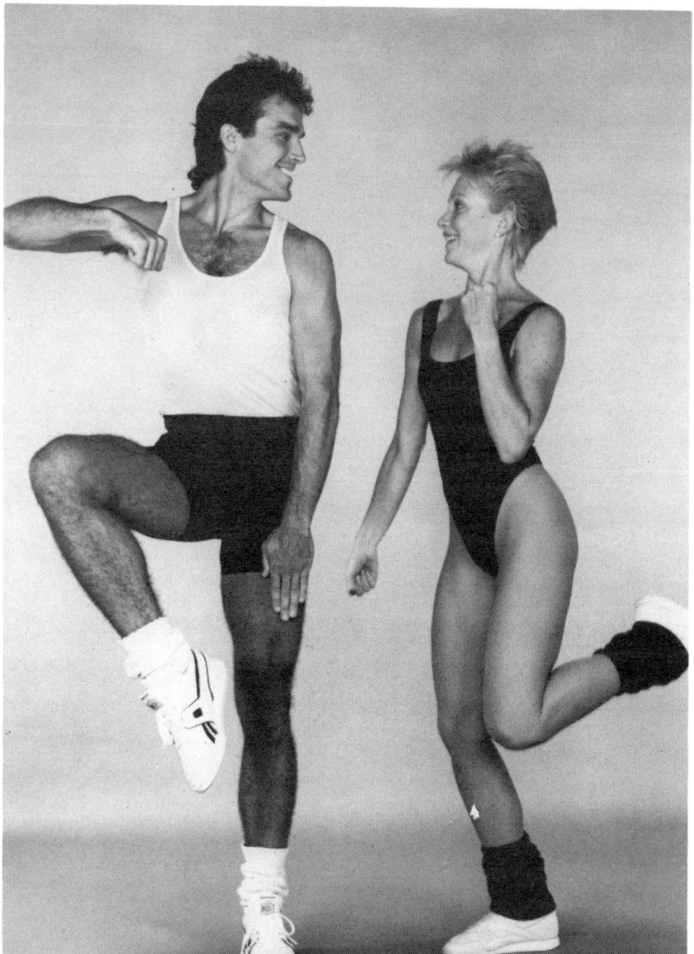

Chapter Three

The Elements of Creativity

Now that we have isolated the moves into their basic forms and explored how to incorporate the elements of variation, it is time to discover how to change the way movement looks and feels. It is here that you will learn how to add the personal nuances that make the movement and the class your own. Anyone, after all, can do a step touch with long lever arms in a low plane. It is *how* you do it, however, that makes the class unique and distinctive.

Before we begin, however, I would like to offer one reminder: even when thinking about creativity and the look of the move, don't forget about the physiological base. You are not choreographing a performance the class will watch, but a series of moves that results in a steady workout. As in every aspect of aerobic choreography, then, keeping the class in the steady state should be the first and foremost consideration.

With that in mind, there are three available elements of creativity at your disposal: design, dynamics and style. As we did with the elements of variation, we will

look at each individual element first, and then integrate them into an effective overall strategy.

Design

Perhaps the easiest way to define design when it comes to creativity is as the shape of a move. If you were to take a Polaroid of the move, what the photograph captures is the movement's design.

When looking at design, all moves fall into two different categories: symmetrical and asymmetrical movements. All movement is one or the other; whether you choose one type over the other depends on a combination of psychological and physiological considerations.

In a symmetrical movement, both halves of the body are doing exactly the same thing. If you were to draw a line from the top of the head down to the middle of both feet, each half would thus be a mirror image of the other. A standard jumping jack with arms moving from the side to overhead, for instance, would be symmetrical, because both halves of the body are doing the same thing. (Figure 3.1)

Symmetrical moves are very useful for several reasons. They impart a sense of stability and balance, and are easy to perceive and to follow. Because they are visually centered, they also have a strong unifying effect on the class. These moves can therefore quickly and effectively pull a class together or increase the room's energy.

They also make excellent transitional steps. When you have finished a combination, you can return to a symmetrical move, use it as your base step and move on from there.

The main drawback with symmetrical moves is that there are not that many of them. High-impact classes can use jumping with the feet together or the feet apart; low -impact classes, bending or straightening the knees

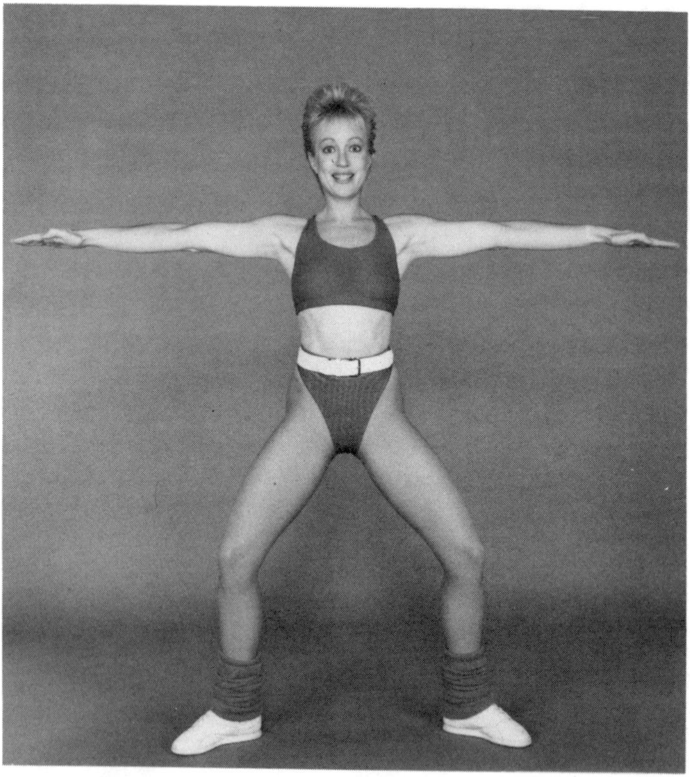

Figure 3.1: *A Symmetrical Move, with both halves of the body mirroring each other.*

with the feet together or apart. Fortunately, although not strictly symmetrical, movements relying on symmetrical arms and simple feet movements can have a similar effect in the workout.

Asymmetrical movement, on the other hand, sees the body's extremities moving in several different directions. Skipping or marching with alternate arms exemplify a simple type of asymmetrical movement. A

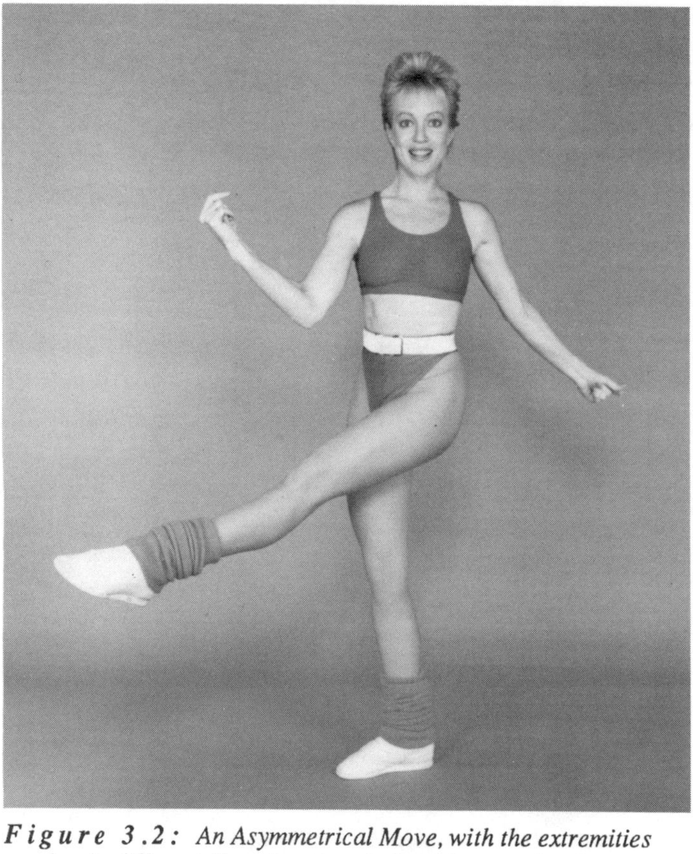

Figure 3.2: *An Asymmetrical Move, with the extremities moving in different directions in relationship to each other.*

pendulum with arms pumping in opposition to the legs is an example of a more difficult asymmetrical move. (Figure 3.2)

When you use asymmetrical moves, you simultaneously release energy in several different directions. Although this can be more difficult at first to perceive than symmetrical movement, it adds an unmistakable sense of adventure, excitement and unpredictability to the class.

Certain types of music lend themselves more to one type of movement than another. Music with a powerful downbeat, for instance, sometimes prompts me into a symmetrical sequence that goes with the beat and makes the song even more powerful. Syncopated music, on the other hand, often is more fun with an asymmetrical movement.

Combining the two types of moves is an excellent way to capture the feel of the music. When putting the combination together, don't forget that people have an easier time perceiving symmetrical movement. The symmetrical movement thus gives their brains a break, and allows both you and them to more easily cue the asymmetrical movement.

A typical combination could include four jumping jacks with the arms opening and closing low, alternated with four skips with the arms alternating over the head. The symmetrical jumping jacks allow the students to mentally ease up a bit, physically prepare for the asymmetrical skips, and visually regroup.

Dynamics

Dynamics, the second major area of creative choreography, refers to changes in how a movement feels. These changes take the form either of tension or tempo.

Tension

Tension can be thought of as a continuum. At one end of this spectrum are sharp, crisp, staccato moves that usually have short levers. At the other are smooth, lyrical, legato movements that usually have long levers. By varying the two types of moves as dictated by the music, you can change the feel of the movement.

To understand this, picture yourself doing a pendulum step, with the legs swinging side to side and letting the arms drop and swing side to side with them in a graceful, lyrical downward arc. Then imagine the same pendulum performed at an increased frequency with a shorter range of motion and a clap on every beat. As you can see, this changes the feeling of the action without changing the basic movements involved. (Figures 3.3 and 3.4)

Another way to visualize tension is by correlating it with the breath's rhythm. You can inhale, suspend the breath for a moment and then exhale in a relaxed, moderate fashion, or your breath can be more like a motor-driven machine, with short inhalations and immediate exhalations. The first rhythm is legato in nature, while the second is staccato.

Songs with strong melodies and weaker downbeats are particularly well suited to the longer legato movements; while funkier songs with pronounced downbeats lend themselves easier to the staccato movements.

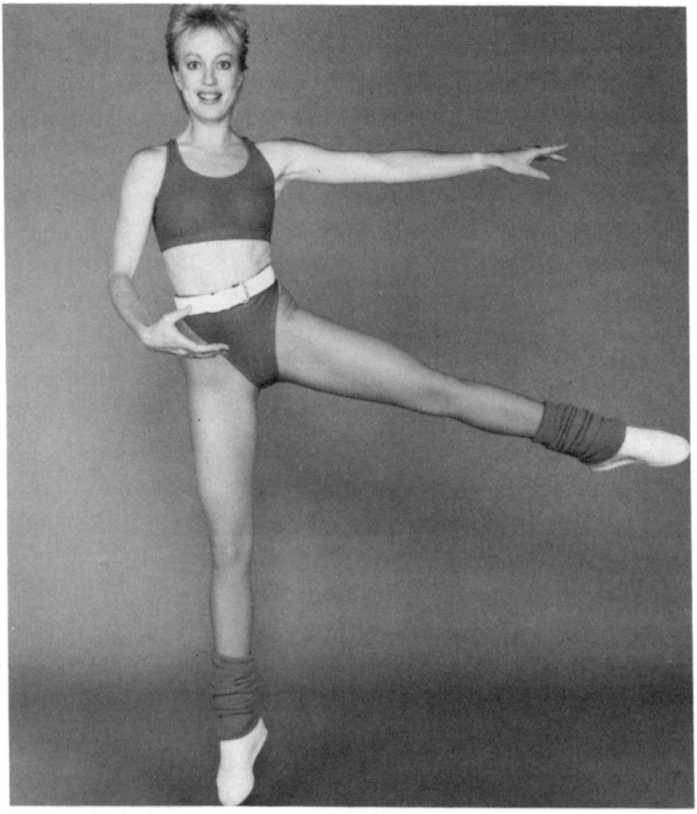

Figure 3.3: *A Smooth, Lyrical Legato Move, with minimal tension and less tempo within the musical phrase.*

Tempo

Despite the popular conception, tempo, the second component of dynamics, has nothing to do with pushing up the beats per minute of the song. Instead it is the measure of how much or how little movement there is in one phrase of music.

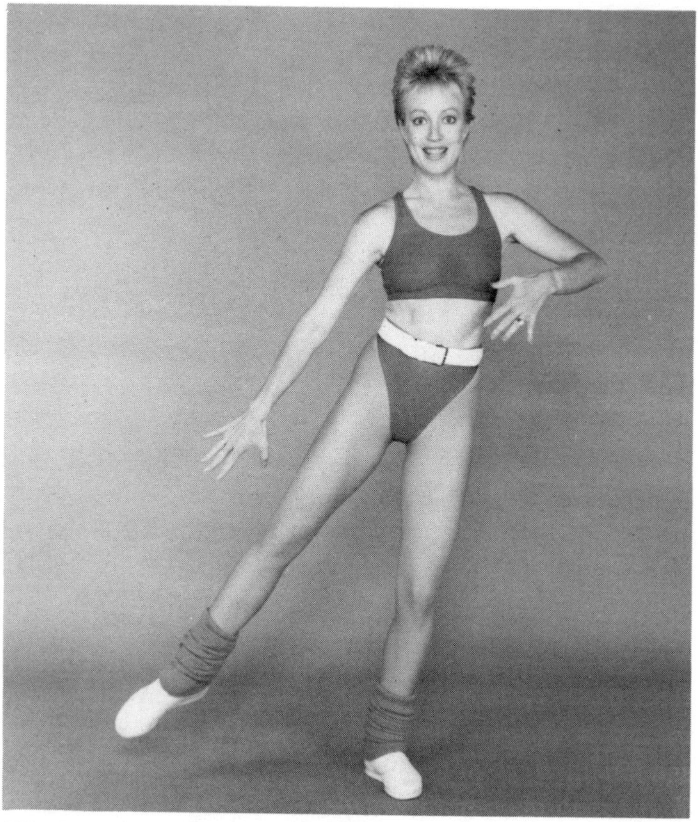

Figure 3.4: *A Sharp, Crisp, Staccato Move, with increased tension and tempo within the musical phrase.*

Generally speaking, tension and tempo are interrelated. Legato movements, which have less tension, tend to result in less tempo within a musical phrase; staccato movements enable more movement and thus more tempo. Usually you increase tension by increasing the tempo, or the amount of movement, within the prhase.

This is a far better way of increasing the energy of a class than the standard aerobic device of turning up the pitch control and increasing the speed of the music. Rather than try to increase the energy of the class in this way, maintain the integrity and aesthetics of the steady state by varying the energy with dynamics.

To understand how you can do this, imagine a four count side to side walk with the arms extended for three counts and dropped on the fourth. Next picture what the move would look like if you move the arms up and down on each beat. Then add syncopation by clapping in a one-two one-two-three pattern. By progressively adding extra movement within the four-count phrase, you have changed the dynamics and energy, and have another tool that gives the move an entirely different feel without changing its basic elements.

Style

Style creates an attitude that fits a piece of music, and is one area in which you can have a lot of fun especially if you move with, not against, the music. There is always more than one way of achieving a physiological steady state. Within that overall guideline, the music it-

self should guide you in this avenue of variation. (Figure 3.5).

Although this sounds obvious, far too many teachers make the mistake of imposing movement on music by filling up the music with the movement, rather than letting the music guide them to the selection of moves.

To avoid that, listen to a new piece of music when you get it, and see how it makes you feel. Go into the

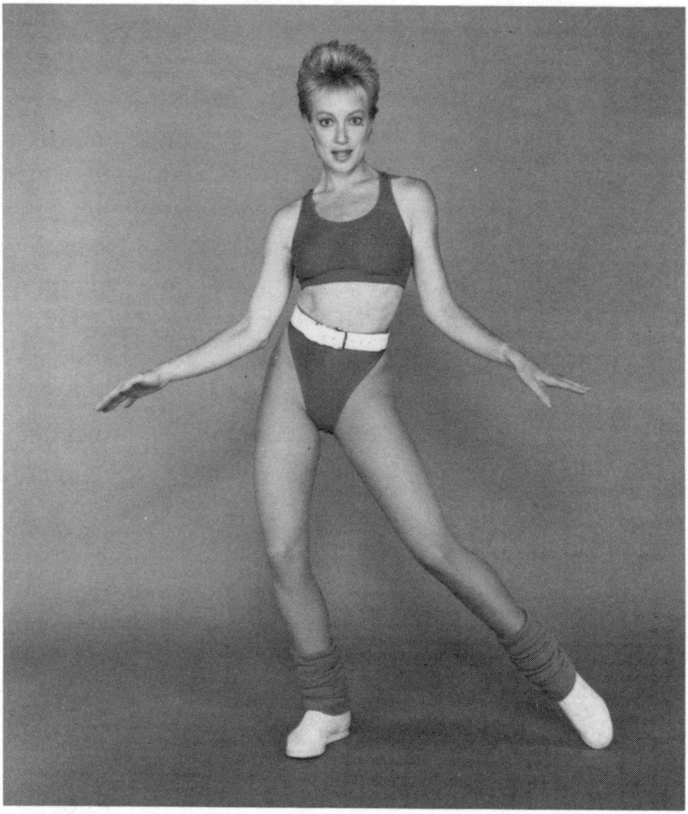

Figure 3.5: *Style, an attitude that makes the move fit the piece of music.*

room by yourself, put it on, and dance to it as if you were at a club. If you were to listen to "La Bamba," for example, you would hear a song with an unmistakable Latin feel, and would probably want to capture that with smooth, gliding moves. A Little Richard song such as "Great Gosh a Mighty," on the other hand, is much more a driving rocker with a 50s feel. I would reflect that with moves such as twisties and with lots of tension and tempo.

To convey the music's feeling in class, I recommend faking established dance steps, rather than trying to teach the actual dance. With "La Bamba," for instance, I don't use to teach them the actual samba or rumba, but instead use variations on walking that look like but are simpler than the real steps. And rather than do a true jitterbug to Little Richard, I use steps that suggest it.

The reason for this is simple: people in class love to feel like they are dancing, but the steps can be too complicated for them. By simplifying the steps without losing the feel, I can eliminate the intimidation of the intricate steps but keep the resulting excitement and all-important steady state.

When putting together your class, keep a rule we learned from the basic elements of variation in mind: especially at first, give them movement that is reduced to its simplest form. Capture the feel of the music with walking steps and varied rhythms, and take your time if you build a combination. If you move slowly enough to bring them with you, they will not feel frustrated and will stay with the movement long enough to feel its unique style.

As you choose the music, also be aware of its relationship to the other songs. Structure the class so that the songs flow into each other by putting the higher energy songs at the end, and the more melodic first. This provides a natural progression and structure that prevents your students from going wild in the beginning but running out of energy by the end.

Putting It All Together

The elements of creativity allow you to use synergy, that phenomenon in which the whole is greater than the sum of its parts, to make your class exciting. When everything clicks, and you throw in the music and movement and your personality and a sense of fun, everything builds into an undeniably energizing atmosphere.

Once you are providing the physiological framework, the best thing you can do for the class, then, is add a sense of yourself. After all, anyone can do a jumping jack, but no one may be able to embellish it the way you can.

To make it and the other moves your own, use music that you like and then let it move you. Don't overanalyze it, and let the music push you around a bit. If you do, you will know how it makes you feel.

Then only use it when it mirrors how you are feeling that day. When you are in the mood for a piece of music, it will do something to you. But if you use something you don't connect with that day, you are not going

to move as easily. And when you are not inspired, your class won't be either.

Drills

Drill #1 — The Symmetry/Asymmetry Drill

Pick one symmetrical and one asymmetrical move. Put them together in a pattern of about four to eight counts each, and see how they feel. This drill will show you how valuable a tool symmetrical movement can be in setting up and framing your asymmetrical move. This is a good drill to practice your cueing, since the symmetrical move allows you time to cue both verbally and non-verbally. Experience how the psychological break of the simple symmetrical move allows you time to mentally prepare for and subsequently commit to the asymmetrical move.

Drill #2 — The Tension/Tempo Drill

Take one movement (the pendulum or a walk, for example), and see how many ways you can vary the tension and the tempo with one song. Then use different pieces of music to inspire you with the same move.

Drill #3 — The Music Drill

Pick a new piece of music and one of the movements you normally use in your class. Then see how you can make them flow together. Start, for example, with a

four count walk traveling laterally. See how you can add the elements of creativity and vary the moves to fit the music.

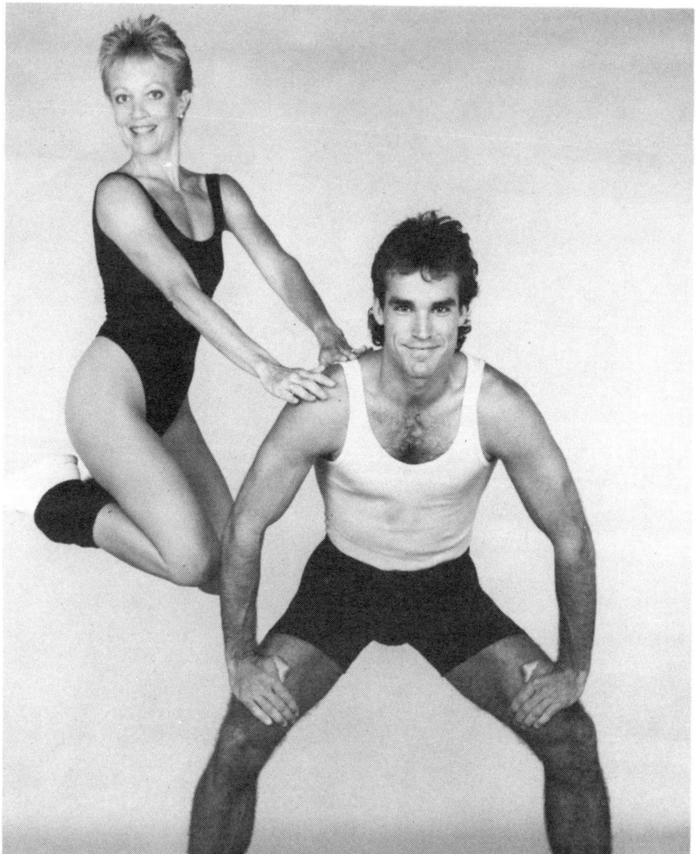

Chapter Four

Achieving Creative Movement

Movement in a Series

We've talked about the individual components of movement, the elements of variation and style. Now it is time to see how to put them together into movement that flows, builds and goes somewhere.

Without this direction, the moves tend to be rushed. When this happens, you usually give away all your steps in the first ten minutes and then have to repeat them over and over for the rest of the class.

If, on the other hand, you learn to take your time and reveal your bag of tricks more gradually, the class will feel that there is always something newer and better coming up. Since the anticipation is as much, if not more, fun than the actual event, keeping them guessing will keep them interested and challenged.

Using what I call movement in a series can create this type of feeling in your class. One way to use movement in a series is by developing a pattern, or circular sequence of steps that is repeated in an unbroken manner.

This device works because the human mind instinctively arranges events into a pattern. If you are using two or four movements that repeat, people will look for the pattern in them anyway. If you give them a clear pattern to focus on, they can relax and more easily anticipate what you are going to do next.

Because the new or less experienced students need more time to learn the concepts, rely on simple moves and patterns first. Then, keeping the basic pattern, vary the movement within it. Take a sequence based on four skips and four knee lifts, repeated for a period of time, for example. By varying the arms, the direction or the rhythm, the class thinks they are doing entirely new movements but in reality are using the same base pattern.

The other type of movement in a series is a linear progression. Unlike patterns, linear movement progresses from one step to another in a seemingly random fashion. It still builds, but does not use repetition in predictable manner. An example of a linear progression could be a step touch with a variety of arm movements followed by a step with a heel dig and then a low cross kick with varied levers and plane of arms to a knee lift, etc.

The best results are usually obtained when you combine the linear and patterned movement. Build a specific pattern, move into a more complicated linear progression using the elements of variation and then

return to the pattern, adding these elements. Or use a linear progression until you develop a pattern.

Start with a step touch with arms in a low plane and build to knee lifts with arms pumping overhead. So far this is linear. But if you then go back to the step touch, for example, you have a combination that has formed the basics of an effective pattern.

Once you get this far, you can go back to the elements of variation, and by changing one of these at a time, develop unlimited combinations of moves to keep the class enthusiastic and surprised. Since you are only changing one element at a time, you don't have to feel under pressure to come up with something completely new all the time.

If I feel like using a pattern of knee lifts and skips, for instance, I can make it different each class by changing one of the lever, plane, direction, rhythm or intensity. I can use long-lever, low-plane arms on the skips and overhead single claps on the knee lifts. Then, in the next class, I might travel back on the skips and forward on the knee lifts and vary the plane or rhythm of the arms.

By reorganizing the basic patterns, you provide a framework that makes the choreography easier for you because it becomes more organized and easier for the class because it gives them something familiar. Then, by adding the style and dynamics we discussed in the elements of creativity, you can fit the pattern to the music, the particular class and to how you are feeling at the moment.

By being able to adapt quickly to an individual situation, you won't have to rely too heavily on a few stand-

ard moves, or teach a class that is does not reflect your own personality or the particular class's need.

Visual Perception

Visual perception is the ease with which your students can perceive and therefore copy and enjoy the movement. The formula is:

Mental consent = physical expression = results

Our aim here is to faciliate that with crisp, clear choreography.

By making sure their eyes or minds can perceive what you are doing and let the bodies copy the movement, you allow the students to fully commit to the move, and to therefore reap the benefits of a workout. If the choreography keeps them scrambling to keep up with you or forces them to slow down so they can figure out the step, they don't work out as hard.

To help your own visualization, imagine what the class looks like from the back of the room. Surrounding the teacher are a core of students who know all the steps and are doing them with abandon. Once you get to the corners and the back rows, however, the movement becomes less synchronized and the pace less intense because the people here must struggle just to follow the steps. They obviously are getting less of a workout than those people who don't have to slow down or worry about what they are doing.

To eliminate this diversity in the room, your physiological goal when it comes to visual perception is the total absence of confusion. If the choreography is clear and you change only one element of variation at a time, you will give the class a consistent underlying rhythm that keeps everyone working within their training range.

If you ignore visual perception, however, you are going to end up with a class filled with "speed bumps." Unclear choreography has the same effect as speed bumps do in a car. Just as you have to slow down to drive over the bump and then build up steam all over again, the sudden break of rhythm in a workout is irritating because it makes you stop and slow down, destroying the steady state.

To drive this bumpiness out of your choreography, think of a good movement as if it were a pyramid. If you stood back and looked at a pyramid, you would see a smooth, straight line. Once you got closer, you would realize that it really was a series of small steps that fit so well that they give the illusion of smoothness. It is this illusion that is the key to good choreography both from a visual and a physiological standpoint.

The way to achieve this illusion is simply by starting with a base move and then varying one element at a time in a slow, even manner. This creates a sense memory for you and your students. As you build on your base step, you have something you can then come back to. This build-and-return pares away any confusion, and is reassuring to the student.

Generally, if you are clear as to where you are going with the choreography, the class will be similarly confi-

dent. If you are just throwing out random moves with no real idea what you want to do with those moves, however, they too will pick up that confusion. But don't worry if you cannot impart that confidence tomorrow — it takes a lot of practice and comfort with the basic steps and elements.

The time practicing is well spent, however, because once you become adept at facilitating visual perception

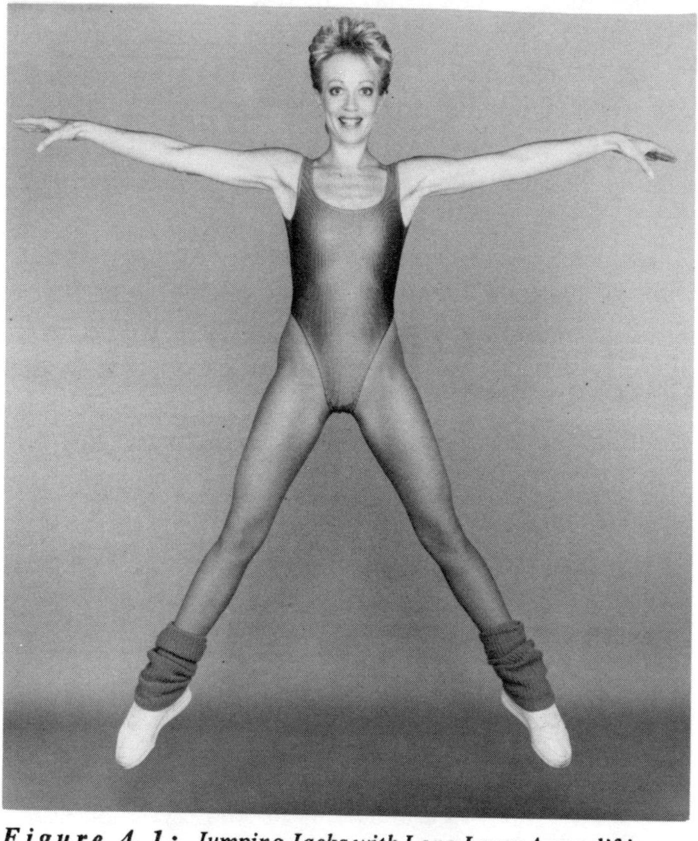

Figure 4.1: *Jumping Jacks with Long Lever Arms, lifting shoulder high and closing to the sides.*

for your students, you will be in a better position to improvise and to enjoy yourself. When you know how to use the elements of variation, you can get from one move to another, say a jumping jack to a knee lift, in four or five steps, keeping them at a steady state the whole time.

This sequence could be accomplished by taking the jumping jack with regular arms (Figure 4.1) to arms

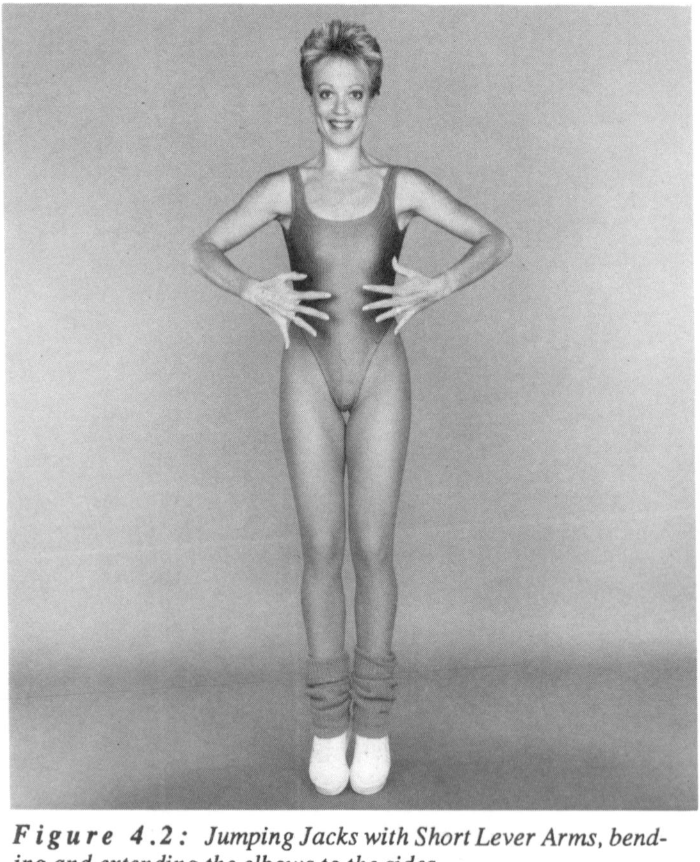

Figure 4.2: *Jumping Jacks with Short Lever Arms, bending and extending the elbows to the sides.*

with shorter levers and the same feet (Figure 4.2). Next raise the arms to the chest (Figure 4.3); then lengthen the lever so that arms cross (Figure 4.4); hold the arms in front and bend them at the elbows so that the fist goes to the shoulders (Figure 4.5); push and pull the arms overhead (Figure 4.6); keep the arms and now change the feet to a jump with the feet together (Figure 4.7); and then, finally, move into a knee lift (Figure 4.8). Be-

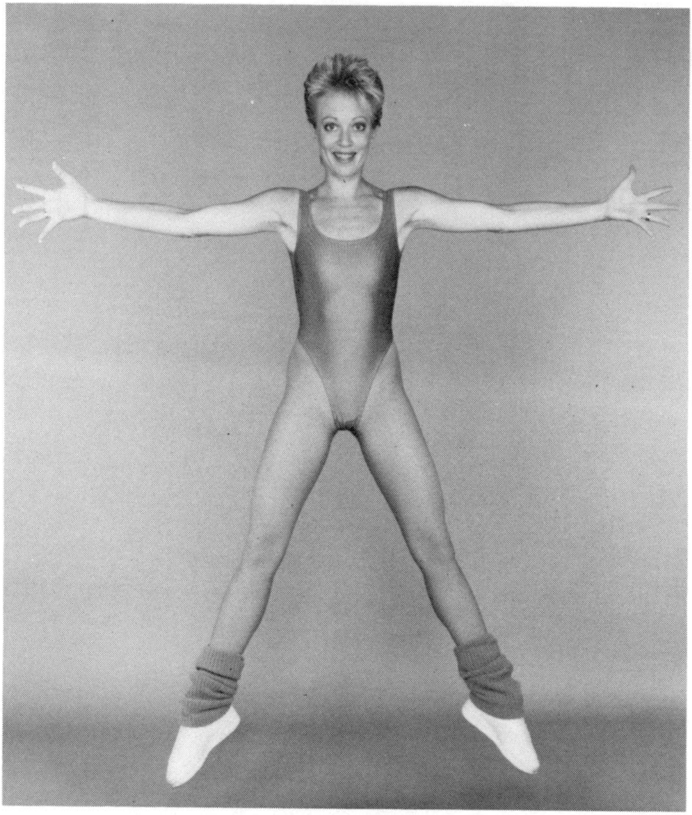

***Figure 4.3:** Jumping Jacks with Short Lever Arms, bending and extending in front of the chest..*

cause this is just one of countless routes you can take to get there, the class need never get boring or unnecessarily repetitive.

You can create good visual perception in two ways. The first is to know where you are going, as with the above example. But a plan is not always necessary. You can also change one element of variation at a time with no end goal other than maintenance of a steady state.

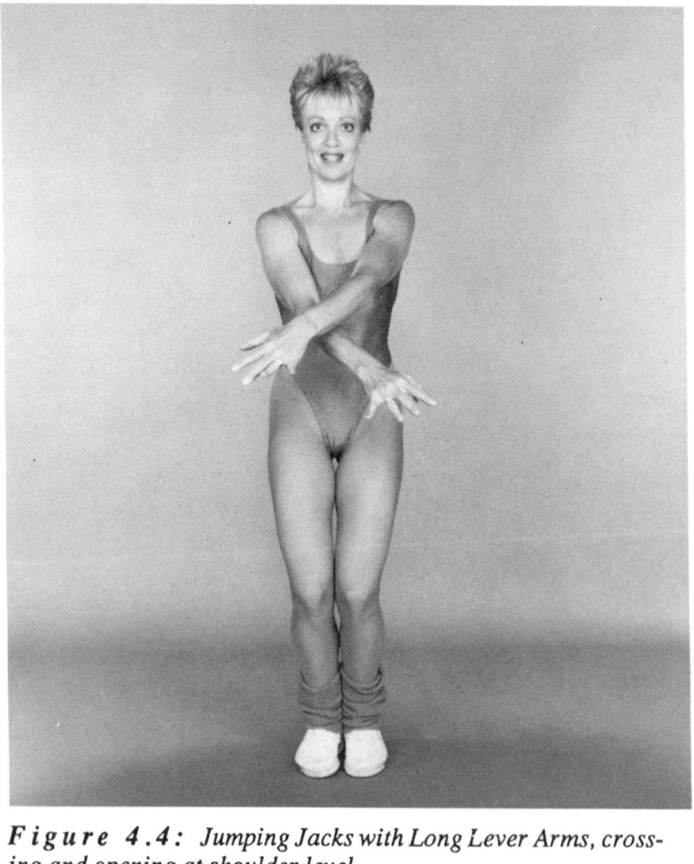

Figure 4.4: *Jumping Jacks with Long Lever Arms, crossing and opening at shoulder level.*

No matter what the moves are, you want to keep the class working in between 65 and 80 percent of their maximal heart rate. If they are not, you can raise the plane or lever, add direction or find another way to add intensity. If the class is at a premature peak, you can bring the intensity down a bit by doing things such as shortening the lever or lowering the plane.

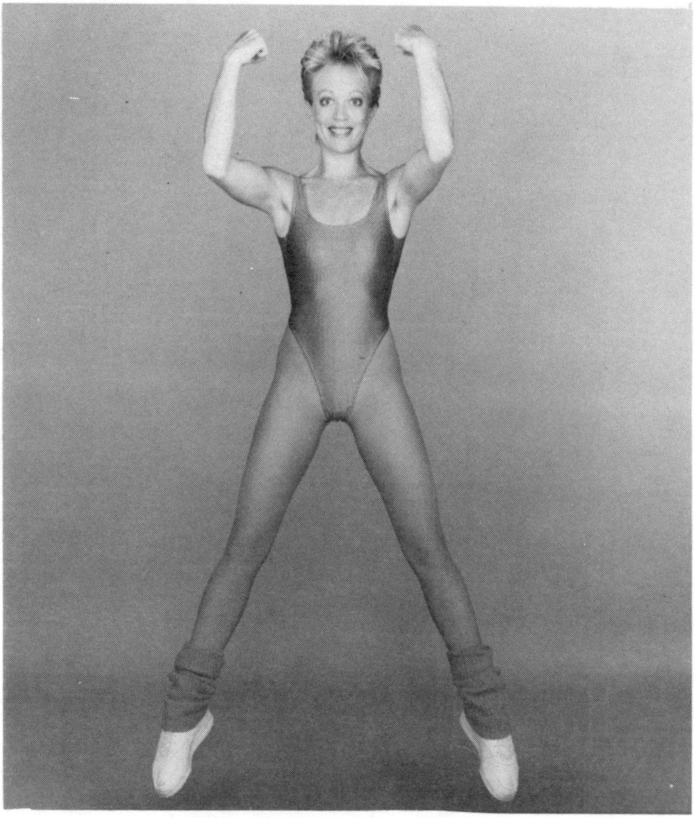

Figure 4.5: *Jumping Jacks with Short Lever Arms, bending and extending in front of the body.*

The whole key to effective choreography then becomes intensity. By choosing your moves according to how intense you want the class to be, you immediately narrow your choices from an overwhelming number to a more manageable selection. By prompting your selection from this consideration, you no longer have any need to pull moves out of a hat.

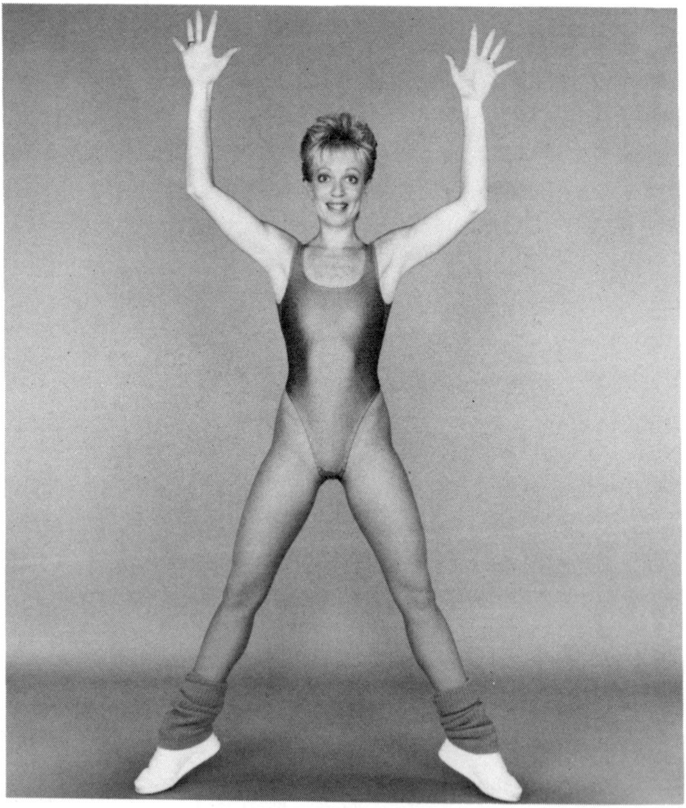

Figure 4.6: *Jumping Jacks with Alternating Long and Short Lever Arms, pushing and pulling over the head.*

By working with visual perception, you arrive at moves the student finds easy to see, easy to do and easy to commit to. In the process, you allow yourself to become a real teacher, rather than someone who forces the movement out in a frenzy.

To become skillful at affecting easy visual perception, you have to become adept at breaking movement down and putting it back together.

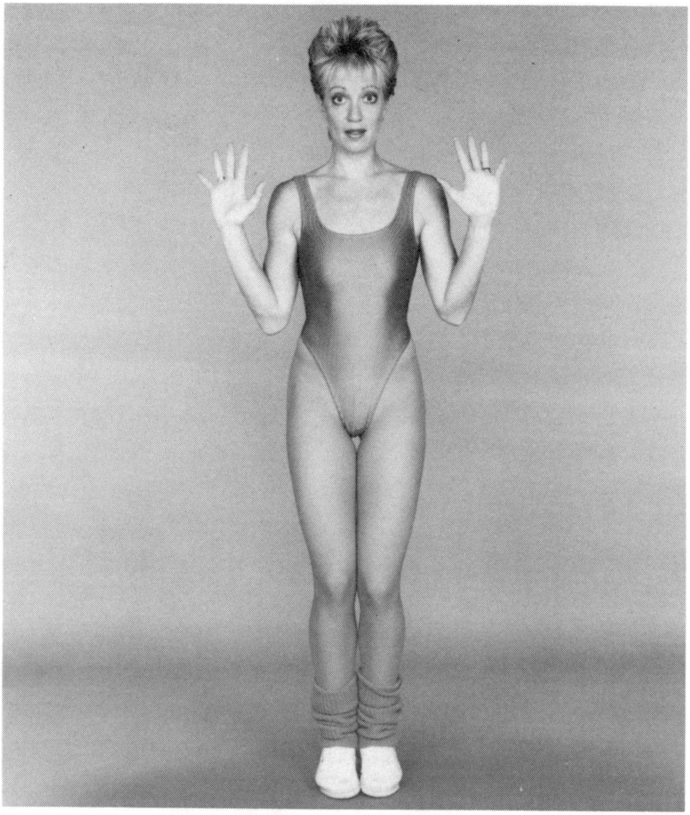

Figure 4.7: *A Jump, with feet together, arms pushing and pulling overhead and then to the sides.*

To develop that ability, pretend you are a stick figure at first. Then show the mechanics of the base step without any style or embellishments. This gives the students a sense memory, and lets them understand the components of the step.. Then add one element of variation at a time. When you do this slowly, the students can develop a cumulative memory that can include up to four or five of these variations.

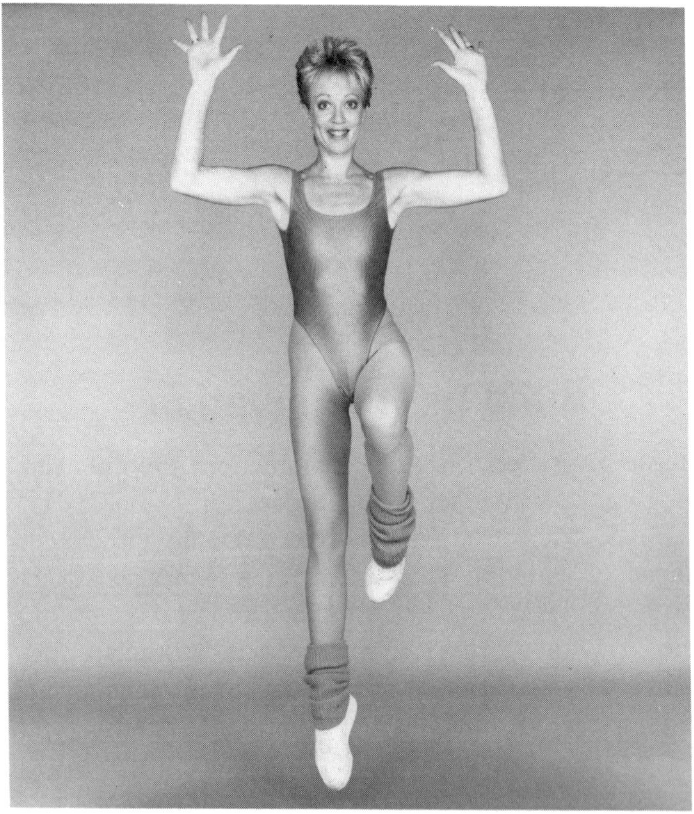

Figure 4.8: *Knee Lifts, with alternating legs, arms pushing and pulling overhead and then to the sides.*

This process can be used in classes of all levels. I believe that students can handle complex moves and patterns, but you have to build to them slowly. Advanced students generally can follow a build faster because they have greater kinesthetic awareness and therefore may need less repititions between the variations. But if allowed, beginners can follow good choreography too.

By building speed according to the class's ability level and varying only one element at a time, the student will be able to move without confusion and to explore his or her own potential for style variation. If they like a move and want to bob their head or shimmey their shoulders to it, for instance, they will feel secure enough to do that and, along the way, have a good time with it.

Building Combinations

Simply stated, building combinations involves putting patterns together. The combination can be as uncomplicated as using one base movement with two elements of variation, such as four counts of a step touch with long lever arms in a low plane and four counts of a step touch with short lever. Or it can be a more challenging combination of two different base steps such as a jumping jack and a skip. A four-count jumping jack with arms pushing and pulling overhead followed by a four-count skip with alternating long lever arms in a low plane would be an example of this.

Our goal in all this harkens back to the goal of visual perception: an easily understood unit of movement that builds momentum while maintaining continuity and the steady state.

There are a few different ways of building combinations that help you maintain a steady state. By building them correctly, peak moves such as jumping jacks in high-impact and lateral moves in low-impact can be

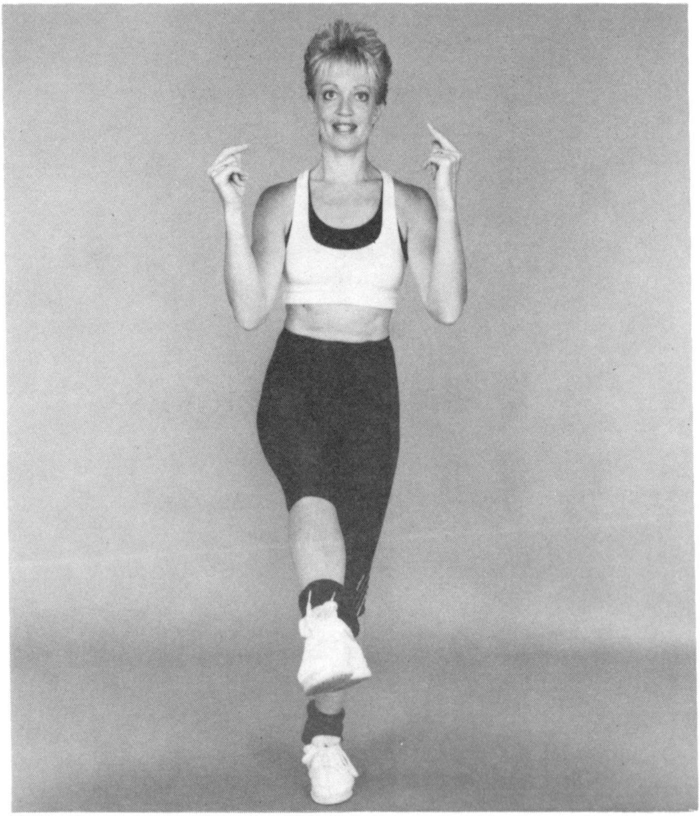

Figure 4.9: *Low Intensity/High Intensity Combination, Part A: a skip and short lever, low plane arms.*

used without forcing the class into anaerobic levels, and without overusing these moves to the point where you are placing excessive stress on the body.

The four ways to build combinations are: low intensity/high intensity; complex/simple; directional/stationary; and low/high impact.

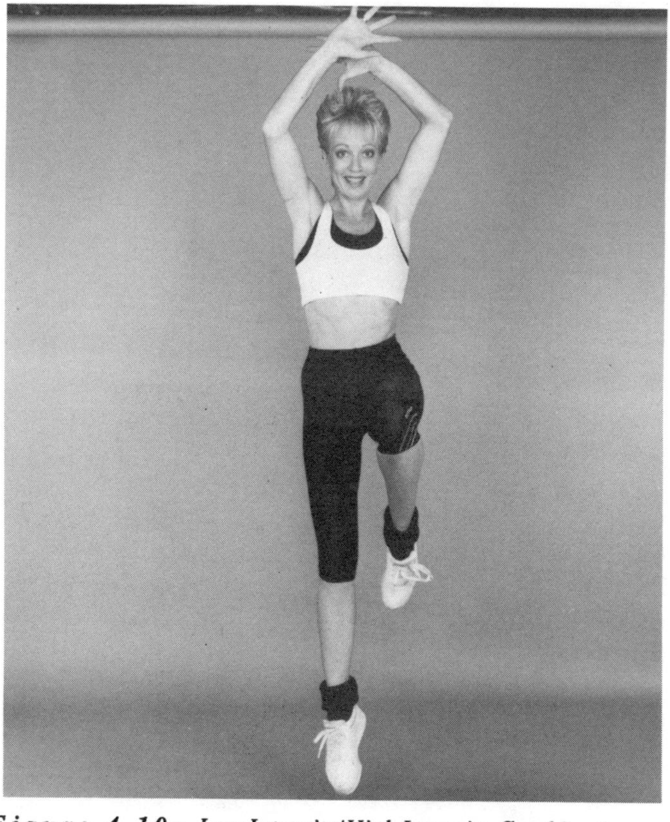

Figure 4.10: *Low Intensity/High Intensity Combination, Part B: knee lifts with arms pushing overhead, then pulling down.*

1. **Low intensity/high intensity combinations.** As its name implies, this is achieved by combining low and high intensity moves. For four counts, for example, skip with short lever, low plane arms (Figure 4.9); and alternate with four counts of higher intensity knee lifts with both arms reaching and pushing overhead (Figure 4.10).

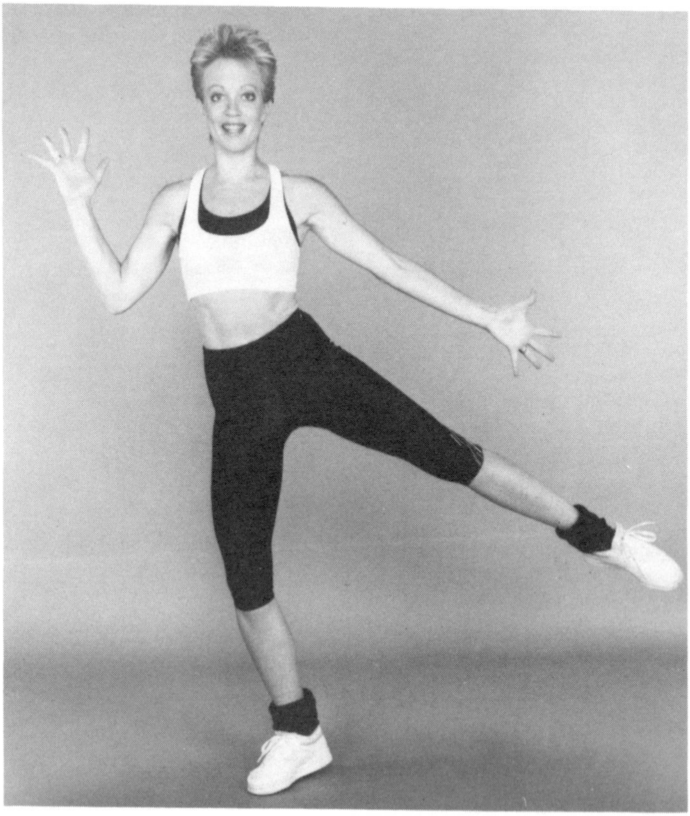

Figure 4.11: Complex/Simple Combination, Part A: a pendulum with short lever alternating opposing arms.

As with the other combinations, I have found that four to eight repetitions of each move is generally a good choice, especially when you are building combinations. By beginning with eight repetitions of each move and working down to four, you can keep the steady state, reduce stress, and keep the action easily perceived without becoming boring. Keep in mind, however, that when you are traveling direc-

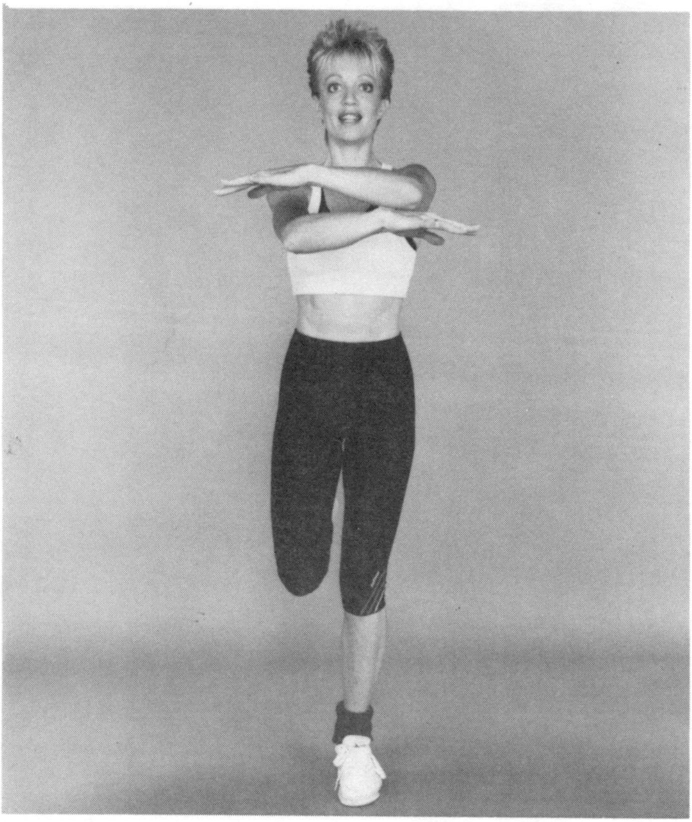

Figure 4.12: *Complex/Simple Combination, Part B: a jog in place with long lever arms opening and crossing at chest level.*

tionally, you probably will run out of room by the eighth count, so you may want to begin with four repetitions.

2. **Complex/simple combinations**. An example of this type of combination is a pendulum with short lever, alternating opposing arms (Figure 4.11) and a jog in

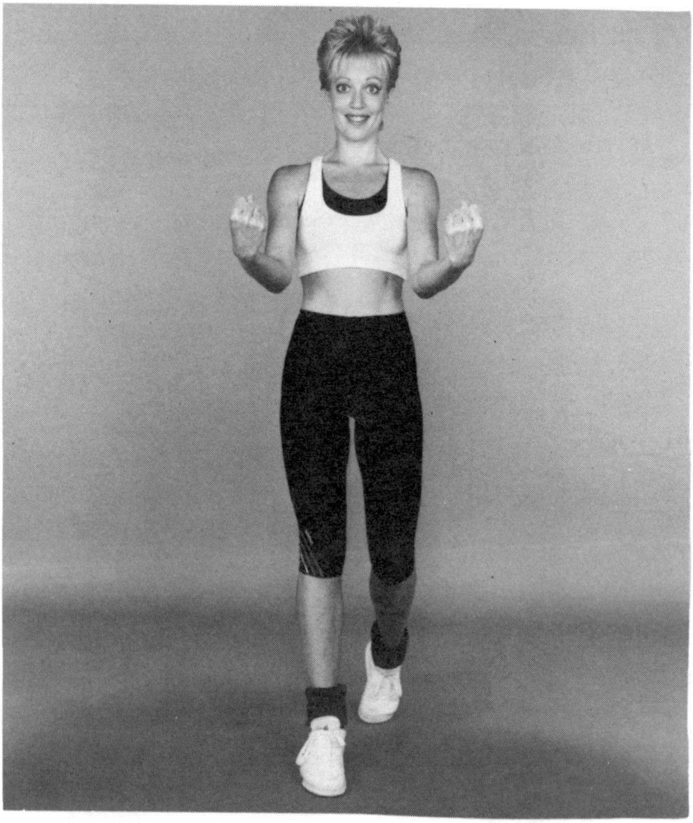

Figure 4.13: *Directional/Stationary Combination, Part A: walk backwards or forwards, arms bending and extending low.*

place with long lever arms opening and crossing at chest level (Figure 4.12).

Usually the complex moves will be of lower intensity because they put more movement into a given period of time and therefore will require shorter levers and a smaller range of motion. These complex movements are also usually asymmetrical in nature. Simple movements are very useful in adjusting the intensity and providing a mental break from the complex moves. The students can use this as a chance to regroup and commit to the more complex move without hanging back or stopping. A symmetrical move would be a good choice here.

3. **Directional/stationary combinations**. Combining directional movement with stationary moves can take the form, for instance, of walking back for four counts, walking in place for four counts, forward for four counts, and in place for four counts. When you are moving backwards and forwards, do short lever bicep curls in a low plane. (Figure 4.13). When you are in place, alternate the arms reaching overhead and to the floor. (Figure 4.14).

   As with the simple moves in the previous combination, the stationary sequence lets them prepare and commit to the more difficult directional moves. It also allows you to reduce the stress of the more demanding steps, such as sudden lateral movement, thereby improving the overall design of the class.

   Because moving in a direction tends to have a higher intensity and frequently is more complex than moving in place, you can maintain steady state by

using simpler arms with directional movement and more rigorous arms with stationary movement.

4. **Low-high impact combinations.** To vary the combination this way, you can, for instance, pick four counts of a high impact move such as jumping jacks with long lever, low plane arms (Figure 4.15) and alternate it with four counts of a push-touch alternating

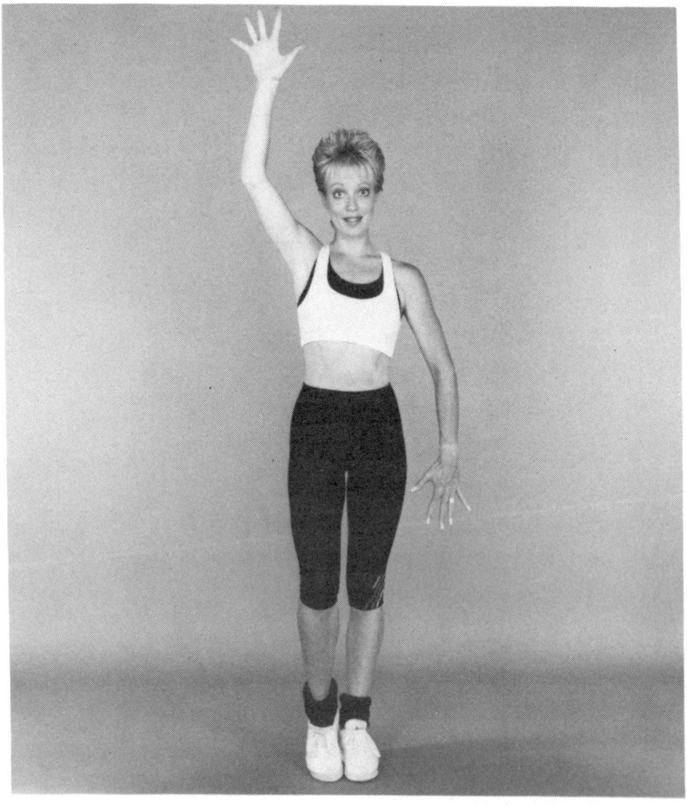

Figure 4.14: *Directional/Stationary Combination, Part B: stationary walk alternating arms overhead and to the floor.*

side to side with the arms in sweeping short levers to one side. (Figure 4.16)

The primary consideration with high and low impact combinations is the reduction of stress caused by high impact moves to the body's musculoskeletal structure while still maintaining steady state. Varying high impact with low impact moves is therefore a hallmark of good contemporary choreography.

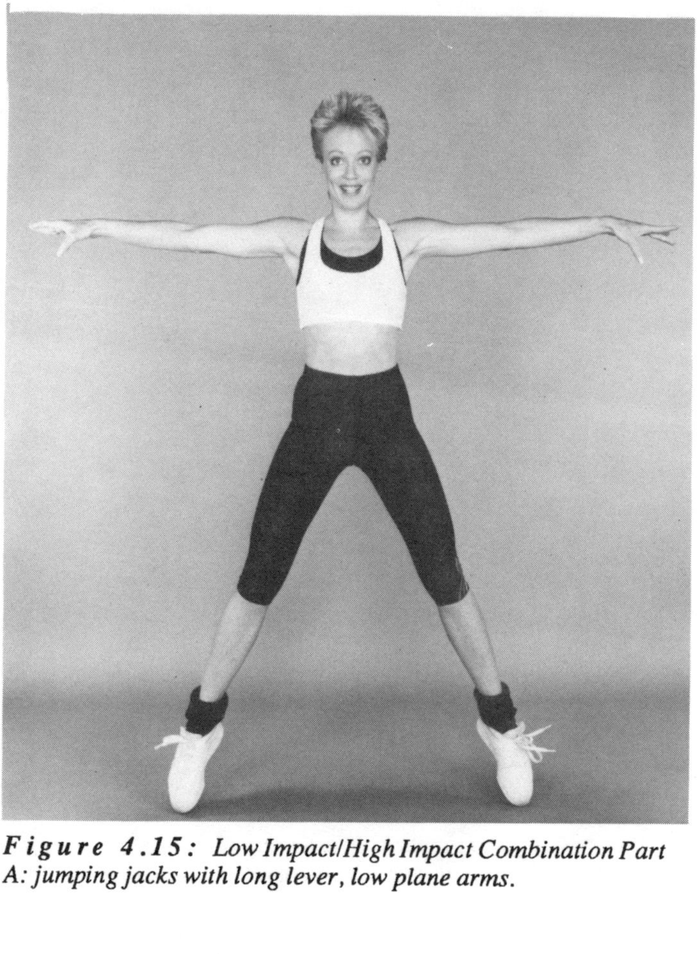

Figure 4.15: *Low Impact/High Impact Combination Part A: jumping jacks with long lever, low plane arms.*

Once you find two moves that fit well together, you can use the elements of variation to come up with so many different combinations that your class need not ever get boring. Because you are using the same basic steps, you are also building the class's sense memory.

Regardless of which device you use, you can end the combination by stripping away all the elements of variation and going back to the original base move. You

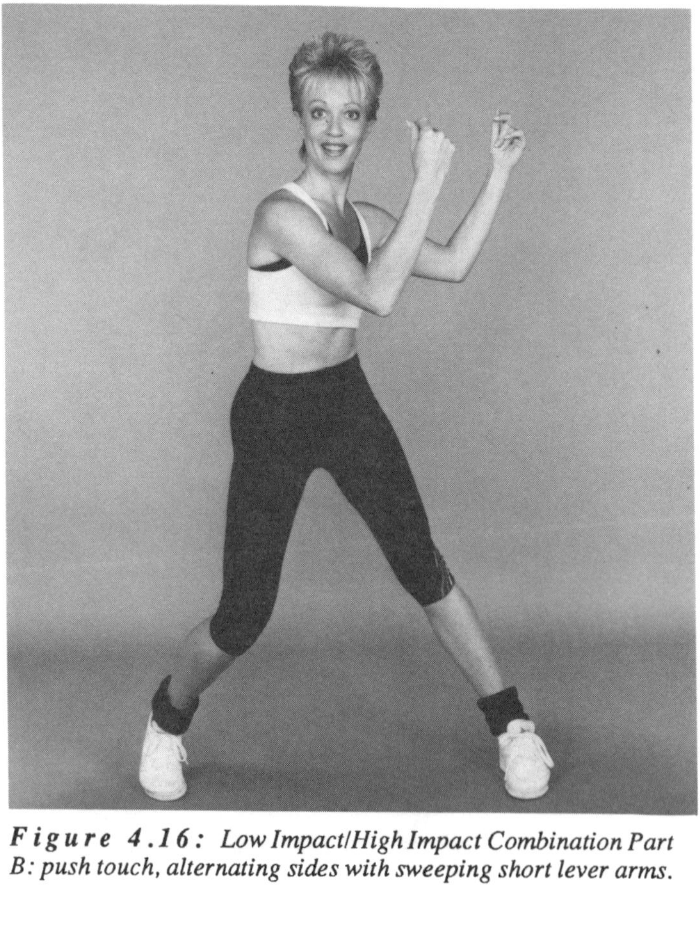

Figure 4.16: *Low Impact/High Impact Combination Part B: push touch, alternating sides with sweeping short lever arms.*

can do this gradually or more abruptly, depending on your next goal and the ability level of the particular class. When you bring them back to the basic step, you let them feel that they have come home.

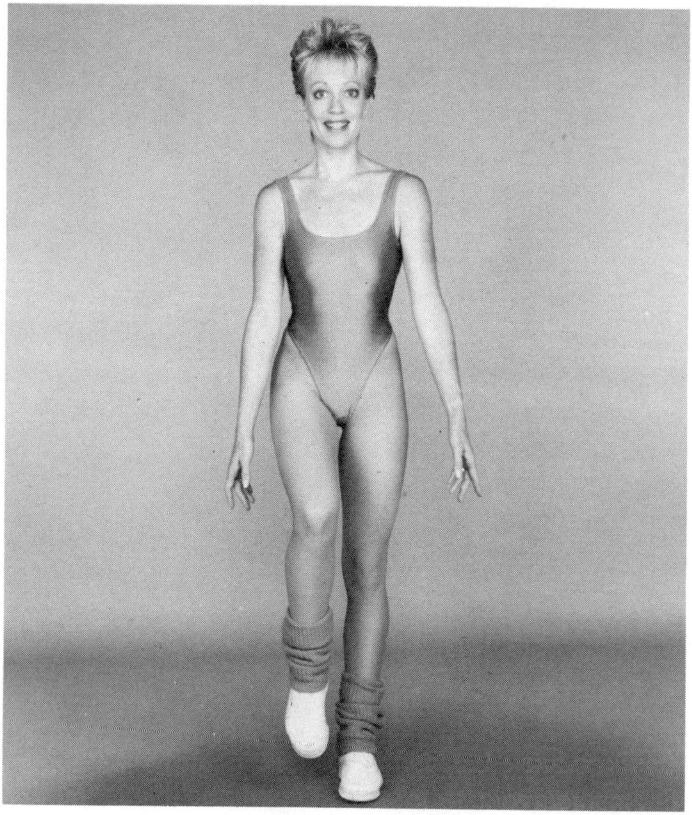

Figure 4.17: *Building Drill, beginning with a walk in place.*

Drills

Drill #1 — The Creative Pattern Drill

Pick one base move. Take each element of variation and then create patterns from that base move. Take a step touch. Use long and short levers to create a pattern that alternates a long and short lever move. With the same base move, create a pattern using two different planes. For example, the feet continue the step touch. The arms could push and pull overhead, and alternate with pushing and pulling at chest level to create a planal pattern.

Using the same base move, find two different rhythmic variations for the upper body. Alternate these back and forth to create a pattern. For example, step touch with a single clap on each touch. Alternate this with a step touch with the arms pumping up and down in a low plane on each beat. By alternating these two different rhythmic variations, you also have added the contrast of sound and silence into your pattern.

Continue in this vein using the elements of direction and intensity to create these same types of patterns.

Drill #2 — The Building Drill

Choose the end product, a four to eight count simple pattern of movmements. Then figure out a base step, and take six to eight steps to build to that destination.

Say, for instance, that you want to get from a walk in place (base step) to a four-count lateral walk with long lever arms circling overhead and ending with a side sweep that repeats to each side.

Step one is a walk in place. (Figure 4.17) Step two could vary the rhythm to a walk two-three with a clap on four. (Figure 4.18). On step three, vary the direction so that you are moving laterally on the walk. (Figure

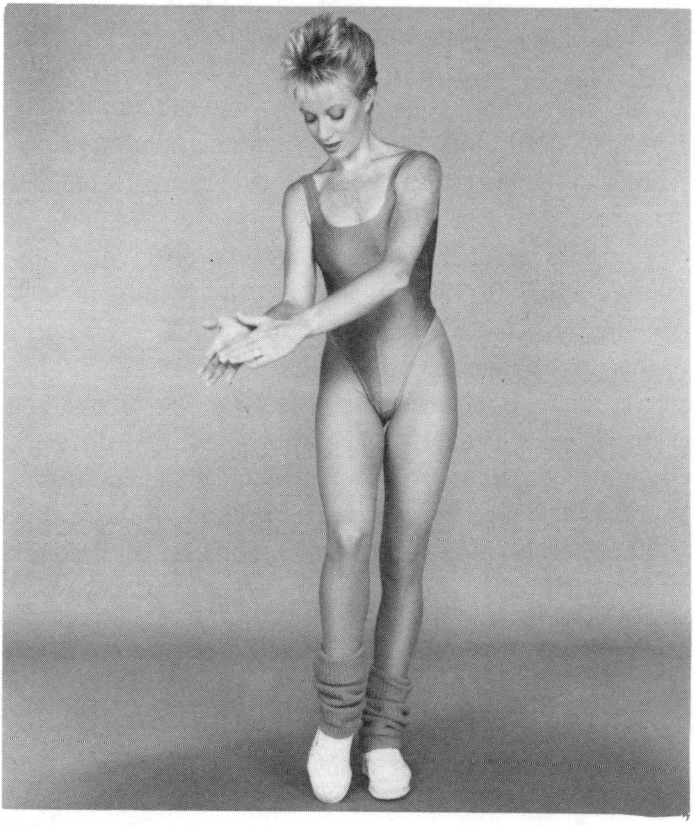

***Figure 4.18:** Building Drill, varying the rhythm with a three-count walk and a touch and clap on count four..*

4.19). Step four varies the arms, adding a short lever bicep curl on four, and arms motionless to the side on the first three counts. (Figure 4.20). Step five varies the rhythm again, and has the arms pumping up and down in a bicep curl. (Figure 4.21). Step six changes the lever, so that the arms extend to a long lever on the fourth count. (Figure 4.22). On step seven, change the plane by adding short lever circles to the bicep curl. (Fig

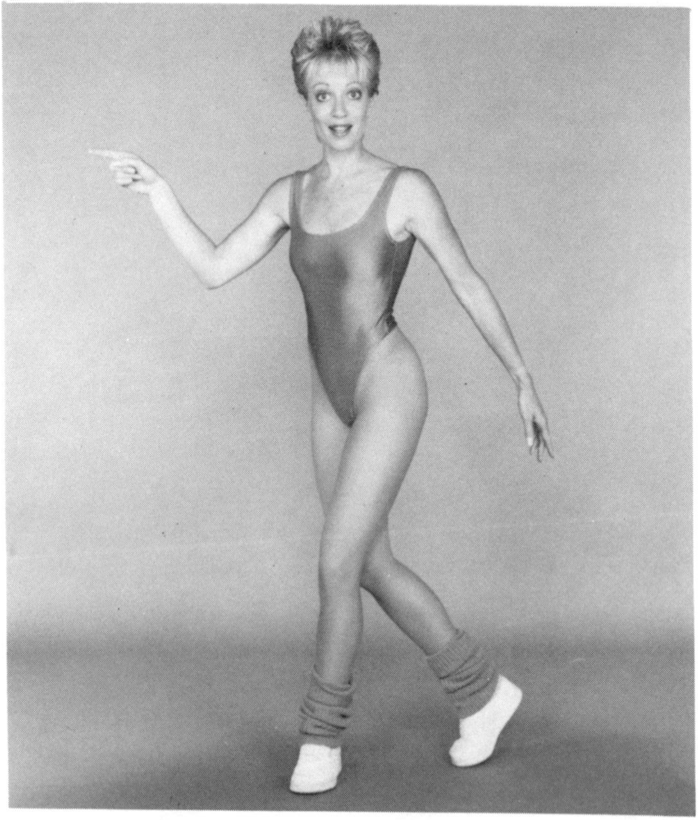

Figure 4.19: *Building Drill, varying the direction by moving laterally with the four-count walk.*

4.23). And on eight, vary the lever, by adding long levers through the full circular motion, keeping the arms parallel to each other. (Figure 4.24).

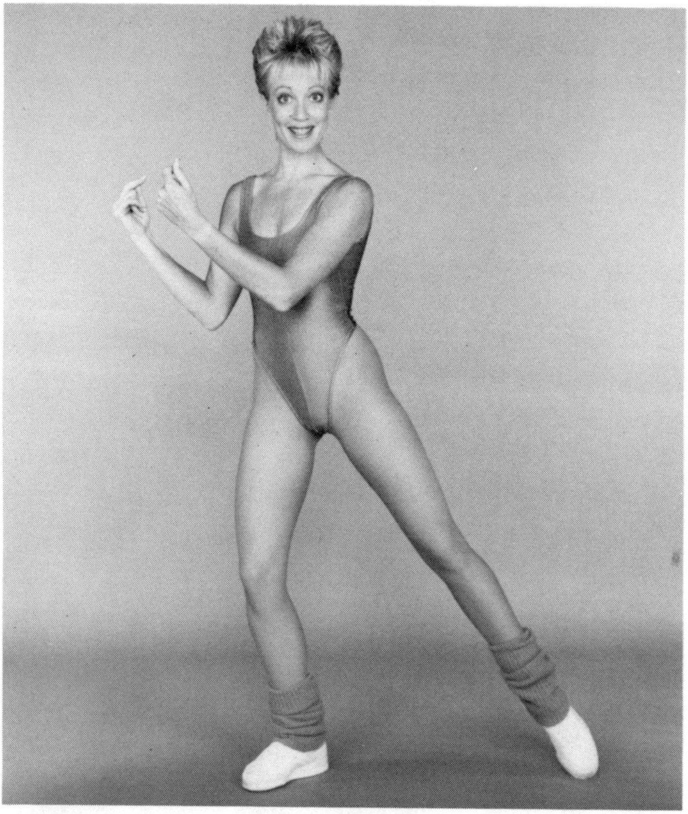

Figure 4.20: *Building Drill, varying the arms as you walk side to side by adding a short lever bicep curl on count four.*

Drill #3 — The Combination Drill

Pick two separate base moves. Choose one of the types of combinations, and put the two moves together. Use a linear progression to develop a pattern. Adjust the pattern to a steady state, and then find the base move that will get you out of it.

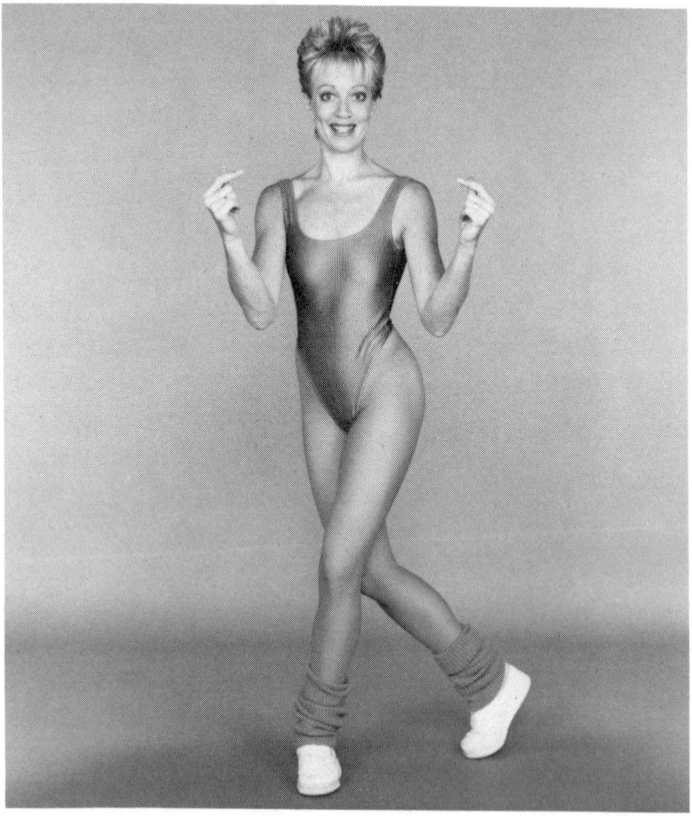

Figure 4.21: *Building Drill, varying the rhythm by pumping the arm in the bicep curl on each count of the music.*

If I choose the step touch as one base move, I would build to a step touch with arms chest level in front pulling back. I would vary the rhythm with two step touches on each side. Then I would vary the direction by facing slightly to the side as I moved laterally. I would then go back to a single step touch, and vary the legs to a knee lift. Next I would vary the plane of the arms to an overhead pull down. Finally I would go back

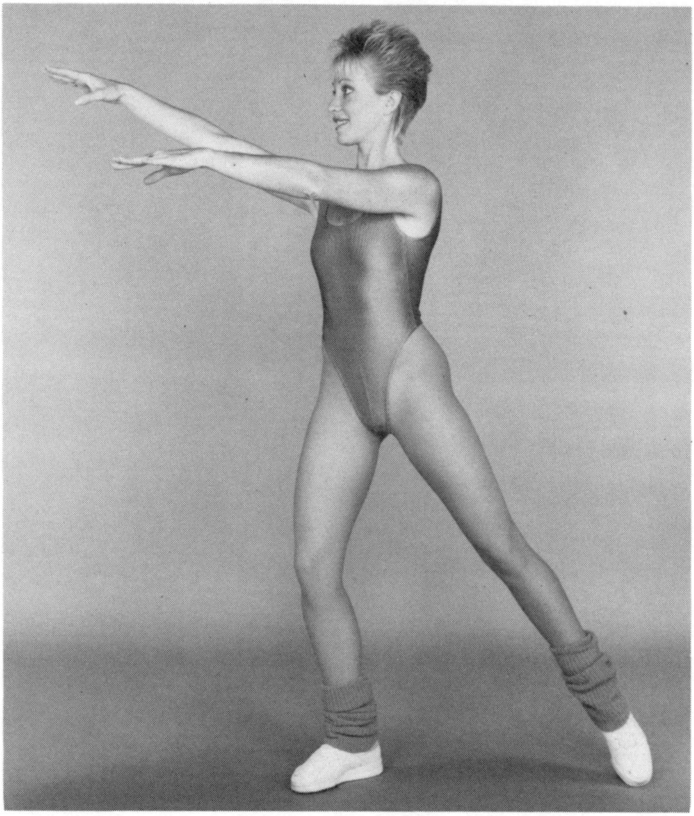

Figure 4.22: *Building drill, extending the arms to a long lever on count four. (Keep short lever bicep curl for three counts.)*

to the double step touch and establish the pattern of a double step touch travelling from one side to the other, and then to four single knee lifts remaining in a stationary position. I would now add the arms, reaching chest high and pulling back on the double step touch, and reaching overhead and pulling down on the knee lifts. This is an example of a directional/stationary combination that should maintain a steady state in your class.

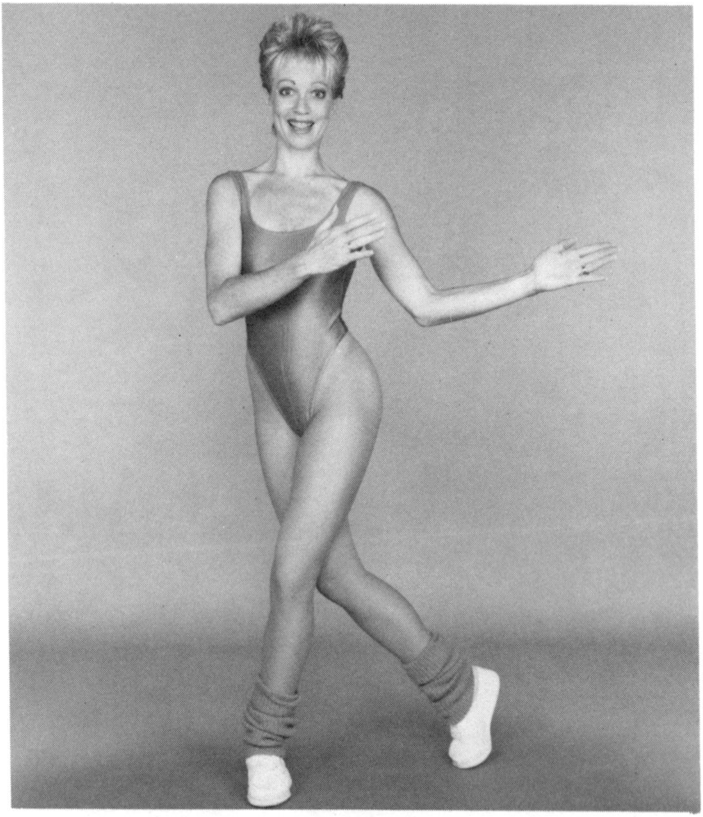

Figure 4.23: *Building Drill, varying the plane by adding a short lever arm circle in place of the bicep curl.*

I would vary the combination by reversing the arms (overhead on the double step to the side; in front of the body on the single); knee lifts; and vary it again by choosing any element of variation dependent on the desired intensity. Then, to regroup, I would take the arms out, return to the step touch, and then build into a walk in place, which is a new base step.

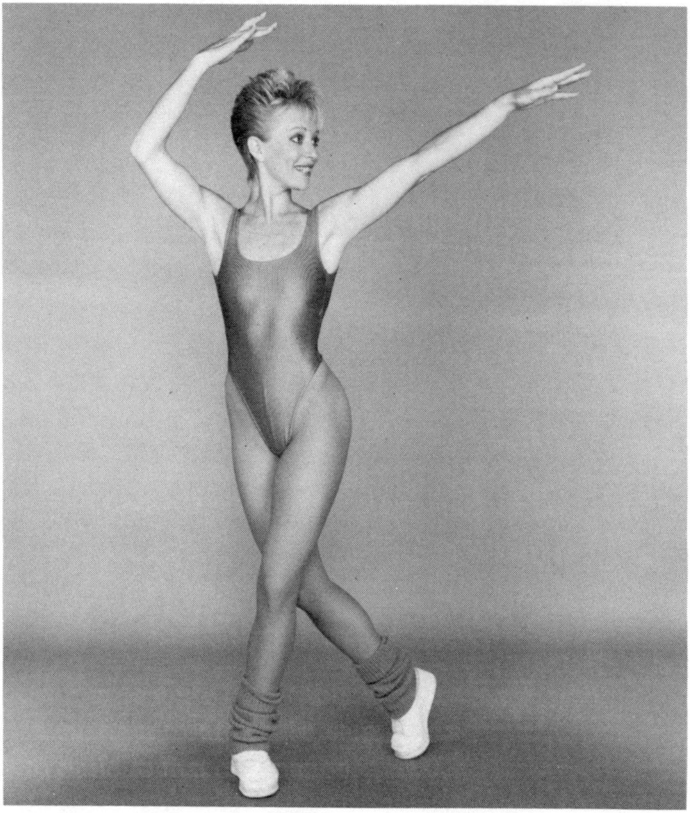

Figure 4.24: *Building Drill, varying the lever by adding a long lever arm circle with arms parallel throughout the circle.*

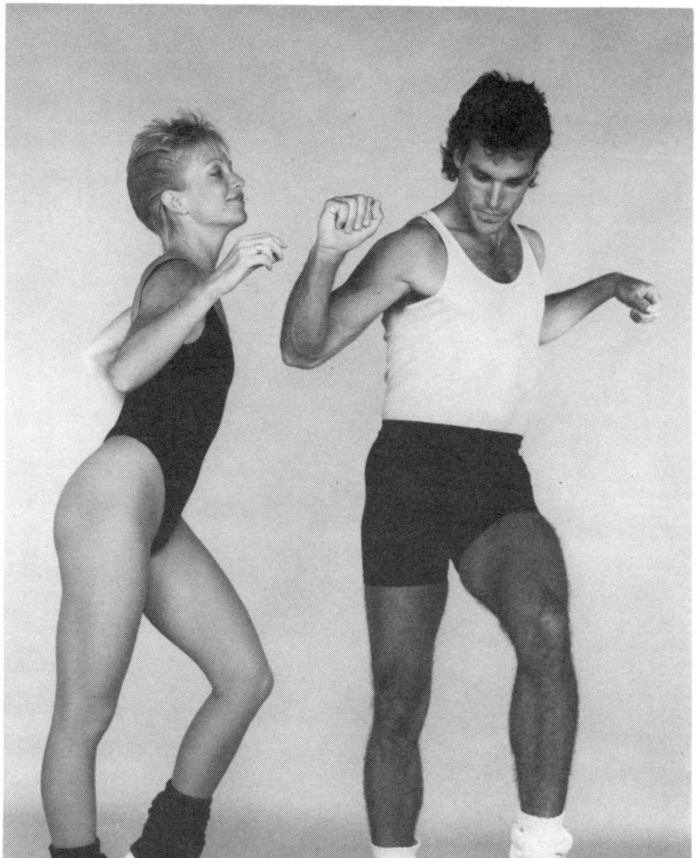

Chapter Five

The Psychology Behind Aerobic Choreography

So far we have concentrated on getting the desired physiological training effects out from your aerobic choreography. For a complete workout, however, you also have to deliver psychological training effects as well. After all, if your class is so repetitive that it becomes a chore or something the student hates to do, they will be far more likely to drop out. But if you can infuse their workouts with a sense of passion, they won't be able to stay away.

This psychological motivation to come back day after day not only insures that the student will build cardio-vascular exercise into his or her daily routine. If you structure the class correctly, however, it also helps them feel successful on an athletic level.

This can happen if they leave class feeling that they have done well in the class. This has less to do with executing every step perfectly, and much more to do with

the realization that they have accomplished something with each move.

For them to do this, you as a teacher have to always remember that no one, even someone who has never been in class before, likes to feel uncoordinated. So a successful teacher takes the pressure off the new students by always teaching to and acknowledging them as well as to the regulars.

If, for instance, you were an overweight beginner coming to class for the first time, I wouldn't expect you to master all the variations and steps, which in fact are there only to keep everyone from getting bored. So rather than feel excluded, you should be made to feel welcome.

I usually do this by explaining to all the students that their goal for this particular class is getting a cardio-vascular workout. The best way to do that, I continue, is simply by staying in motion for the cardio-vascular segment of the class and getting a feel for the movement. Because your goal for the day is maintaining this movement, you not only benefit physiologically from a cardio-vascular standpoint but avoids the intimidation of trying to keep up with more experienced students. When you leave, it will not be with frustration, but with the emotional satisfaction that comes from doing something right.

One way that you can help students feel that way is by correcting them constructively, taking care to point out what they are doing right as well as what needs improvement. I usually begin a correction by acknowledging their command of the basic step. Then I explain that I am increasing the stakes, be it by getting them to

reach into their upper aerobic levels more or by fine-tuning technique. By letting them know I think they are ready for more, they relax with the challenge, commit to their performance and build physiological and psychological effectiveness into the workout.

The whole key, then, is to challenge them physiologically without thrwarting them with too much psychological pressure. The variations should be intellectually stimulating, of course, but the base moves and overall design of the class should not be difficult to the point of confusion. If it is, the students don't work hard enough to get their heartrate into the submaximal zone and leave discouraged.

Since only the rare student will go back to a class three or four times in the hopes of getting the hang of it, preventing this negative reaction is important for both personal and commercial reasons. Our business relies on hooking the student from the first time; having them walk out feeling like a failure is not likely to do that.

Having them leave feeling good about themselves also helps you feel successful. And your feelings of psychological success are every bit as important as your students, because ultimately your class reflects your own self-image and feelings.

I have found that teachers who are psychologically successful are those who achieve consistent low-stress teaching. They don't have to worry about what they are going to do next, but know where they are going and are comfortable enough with that direction to communicate it directly to the students.

There is only one way to achieve this type of success, and there's nothing magical about the solution. It simp-

ly is practice, and lots of it. Dancers know that you can't just perform but have to constantly work on technique and improve it. Teaching is the same way.

Although a good teacher always makes the process look smooth and easy, no one can always think on the spot. Rather than rely on pulling something out of the air, the best teachers know that there is no substitute for spending one to two focused hours a week on your feet by yourself practicing moves and putting combinations together. By doing so, you can enter the classroom relaxed and in control, and devote your in-class time to your students, rather than to the panicked need to pull a move out of the hat.

Don't think of these practice sessions as torture or drudgery, either. They are the only way I know you can develop new moves and combinations, which in turn are the best way to keep yourself involved. When you throw in one new step, variation or combination each class, you have to pay attention to how you are going to get into the variation and out of it, and how the class is going to respond.

This response increases their involvement as well, because it adds to their anticipation. They like the suspense of something that is different enough to be fun but manageable enough to handle. This expectation sets up an exchange of information that reinforces the bond between you and them, and helps your teaching stay in the moment, attuned to the needs and desires of that particular class on that particular day.

I regard practice, then, as part of the equation:

Discipline = Freedom = Personal Style

By learning and practicing your craft, you are free to create and take your routines farther. This pushes you into your own personal style, instead of one that is merely imitative. Then, when as we all do, you sense the beginnings of burnout, you return to discipline and practice so you can recapture your creativity. Soon, as you lose yourself in the music and come up with one or two new touches, you will regain control over your mood.

This evolution, incidentally, does not mean getting wilder and wilder. Instead, the whole point is to hone your skills so that you can get the exact physiological response from the move you choose. And, again, that only comes with and from practice.

This admittedly is not the easy route. But it will take your teaching into a whole other realm. You, like the student who comes in day in and day out, have to be passionate enough about your teaching to want to spend the extra time getting better. If you do, you not only will fulfill your responsibility as an educator by giving the students the means and knowledge with which to achieve mental and physical fitness. You also will be giving yourself the courage not just to get behind the wave and watch someone else have all the fun making up routines. Instead you will be able to jump in and ride that wave first and fastest. And when all is said and done, doing that responsibly and intelligently is the bottom line.

Happy teaching!

Appendix

Choreography and Combinations

1. Base Move: Step Touch

Build: Arms bend and straighten with finger snap at lowest point. Legs vary to heel touch in front. Add crossover heel touch. Arms vary to low diagonal cross-over (across extended leg). Add hand clap on crossover. Vary arms to mid-chest level, then overhead. Arms extend to long lever as they sweep overhead, then bend at the elbow as they pull to one hip. Add knee lift with a slight crossover. Elbows pull to the outside of the lifting knee.

Combination: Four heel crossovers with hands clapping low to outside of leg, then four knee lifts with arms sweeping overhead, then elbows pulling to one hip. Add directional variation by moving back on the heel crossovers. Stay in place on knee lifts, move front on heel crossovers, in place on knee lifts. Vary again by

moving back on heel crossovers, then front on knee lifts, vary again by reversing the arms to overhead sweep on heel crossovers, then low clap to the outside of the lifted knee.

2. *Base Move: Walking in Place*

Build: March in place four times, then move back four times. March in place again four times, then move forward four times. Pump arms on each beat low (in front of thighs). Add overhead push, pulls on the march in place. The finished pattern is march in place four times with arms pushing and pulling overhead; march back four times with arms pumping low; repeat in place and moving forward.

3. *Base Move: Walking in Place*

Build: Walk laterally to either side four times, with a touch on count four. March in place four times facing front. Repeat the step, cross, step, touch to the other side. March in place four times. The arms push and pull overhead as you move laterally. Add a clap, if you want, on the touch at count four. Arms pump low (in front of the thighs) as you march in place. The finished pattern is walk to the side four times with the arms pushing and pulling overhead; then march in place four times with the arms pumping low. Repeat to the other side.

Combination: Walk back four times with arms pumping low; march in place four tiomes with the arms

pushing and pulling overhead. Walk front four times with arms pumping low; march in place four times with arms pushing and pulling overhead. Walk side four times with arms pushing and pulling overhead; march in place four times with arms pumping low. Repeat to the other side; repeat entire combination. Add variation by using rhythm changes such as clapping instead of pumping the arms. Alternate arms instead of pushing and pulling symmetrically.

4. Base Move: Push Touch

Build: Begin with feet apart, shoulder distance. Rock side to side. Gradually favor the rock to one side. Add a heel lift (rock easily onto the tip of the toes) on the favored side. Gradually vary the direction until you are facing one side (foot that is rocking is now the back foot). Gradually change the rock back and forth to a touch then push back (your front foot should now be the moving leg). Add a bicep curl, low with the arms. Vary the plane of the arms by lifting the elbows to shoulder-high on the curl. Vary to a push, pull with the arms slightly above shoulder level. Keep the arms going and slowly vary body direction until you are facing front. The working leg is doing a push touch, with the arms pushing and pulling overhead. Keep the arms going and vary the feet to a twist. Arms vary to alternating arms overhead. Vary to a side-to-side twist with arms at chest level. Vary the feet back to a side-to-side rock. Gradually lower the plane of the arms to a low bend and straighten. Take all movement out of the arms and keep

the side- to-side rock going. Repeat the entire build from the beginning by now favoring the opposite side. The build can be extended by adding variations during the twisties such as lever and planal variations with the arms.

5. Base Move: Twisties (High or Low-Impact)

Build: Twist in place with the feet about shoulder distance apart. Add alternating arms (short lever) at hip level. Gradually lift arms overhead, pulling elbows to hips. Then build to long-lever alternating arms. Vary the rhythm by adding double count twisties (two bounces or steps on one side), keeping the arms long lever. Vary back to single count twisties with the arms changing to short lever and the knees bending slightly.

Combination: Double twisties (two bounces or steps to each side) four times with the arms alternating long lever. Single twisties eight times with the arms alternating short lever. Build down to doubles twice, then singles four times. Add directional variation by staying in place on the doubles, then moving to the side on the singles. Additional variation can be achieved by using different arm patterns such as symmetrical arms overhead and down on the doubles, and arms opening and closing at chest level on the singles.

6. Base Move: Step Touch

Build: Step touch with the arms reaching out at chest level in front and pulling back (fist to hips, elbows behind the body). Build to two step touches on each side. Vary the direction by facing slightly side as you move laterally. When the pattern is set, come back to singles and vary the plane of the arms by reaching overhead and pulling down.

Combination: Double step touch to one side with reaching and pulling arms at chest level. Repeat to the other side. Face front with four single step touches, arms reaching and pulling down overhead. Vary the combination by reversing the arms (overhead on doubles to the side, in front of the body on singles). Vary again by adding alternating arms on the singles, and either high or low plane arms on the doubles (depending on the desired intensity level).

7. Base Move: Jumping Jacks

Build: Begin with double-count jack (two jumps feet out, two jumps feet together). Add arms, opening side then crossing low in front. Increase intensity by reaching overhead as feet go out, double clap in front as feet are together. Build to single jacks with arms opening and closing side and front.

Combination: Two double-count jacks with arms overhead, then clapping in front. Then four single jacks with arms opening and closing side and front. Repeat

two doubles, then four singles. May be combined with the following series:

8. Base Move: Skipping

Build: Skip with legs reaching front. Add symmetrical arms, starting low at the sides and reaching straight front. Arms stop at shoulder level. Vary the plane of the legs by extending them side. Arms change to side reaches (jumping jack arms).

Combination: Eight skips front with arms reaching front, then eight skips side with arms reaching side. Build down to four on each side. Arms may be varied by adding long or short lever outward circles on the side skip or by adding overhead push pulls on the front skip.

Four Part Combination: Two double-count jacks as in the above combination with four single jacks. Repeat. Add four skips front as above, then four skips side. Repeat the entire combination. Add directional variation by moving to the back on the first set of double, then single jacks. Stay in place for the second set of double, then single jacks. Move forward on the front skips, then stay in place on the side skips. Repeat the entire combination adding elements of variation with the arms, or by varying the rhythm (two of each move).

9. Base Move: Lunges

Build: Begin by jumping in place, then into a jumping jack. Vary the direction to a diagonal lunge. Arms begin with one arm sweeping long lever from hip to overhead; then add both arms together. Alternate single lunges side to side.

10. Base Move: Knee Lift

Build: Begin with single knee lifts one on each side. Arms are the same as on the above lunges.

Combination: Combine four knee lifts with four lunges, alternating singles side to side. Add directional variation by moving back slightly on the lunges and forward on the knee lifts.

11. Base Move: Jumping with Feet Together

Build: Jump side to side in a skiing motion. Arms move with the legs, one extending long lever directly out to the side, the other extending short lever across the body in the same direction. Build to a jumping jack with both arms extending out to the sides (basic jack arms).

Combination: Jump side to side four counts with arms moving with the legs. Add four jacks with arms out to the sides. Repeat four counts each.

Four-Part Combination: Jump side to side four counts; add four jacks; add four knee lifts; add four lunges. All arms are the same as above. Add directional

variation by moving backwards on the side-to-side jumps. Stay in place on the jacks. Move forward on the knee lifts, and stay in place on the lunges. Repeat the entire combination. Add variation by changing the long-lever arms to short levers, and the low planes of arms to high (overhead) planes.

12. Base Move: Walking in Place

Build: Begin walking in place. Then add a three-count walk with a touch and clap on count four. Repeat, then begin to add slight movement to the side. Continue the progression, ending with strong lateral travelling side to side. Vary the touch on count four to a knee pull. Arms vary from a clap on count four to a pull in with the elbows to the hips. Add a push pull with the arms (arms are either pushing or pulling at shoulder level on each count). Change the plane of the arms to overhead pushing and pulling.

13. Base Move: Push Touch

Build: Push touch four times on each side, facing front. Arms build to upright row and push down (in front of the body). Vary the direction by facing slightly to the side (shoulders, hips, knees, toes lined up). Arms vary to single arm lift and push (front arm moves, back arm rests on thigh for support). Change the plane of the arms to chest level push, reaching diagonally across the

body. Vary the rhythm by building down to two push touches on each side, then singles on each side.

Combination: Walk four counts to one side with a knee pull on count four. Add two push touches with the same leg that the knee pulled. Repeat to the other side. (The rhythm is walk, walk, walk, pull, push, pull, push, pull...repeat.) The arms push and pull at chest level on the walks, and one arm reaches and pulls in on the push touches. Vary the direction by turning slightly to the direction you are travelling. The push touches face side (front leg and arm are moving). Vary the intensity by reaching and pulling overhead on the walk, and both arms push, pulling on the push touches.

The same combination can be done with directional variation by facing front with jumping jack arms on the walk, and short lever overhead circles on the push touches. This combination can also travel forward and back as well as laterally. Combine forward and back travelling with lateral travelling for a four-part combo.

Index

See Reverse Side

for Ordering

and Seminar

Information!

ORDER FORM

MOVES INTERNATIONAL
1849 Sawtelle Blvd.
Los Angeles, CA 90025
(213) 454-7490

Please send me _______ copies of *MOVES, The Foolproof Formula for Creative Choreography* at $15.95 each. I enclose a money order or check to "Moves International."

________ books at $15.95 each ____________

Shipping at $1.50 for the first book and $1 .00 for each additional book ____________

Californians only: 6.3% sales tax ($1.00 per book) ____________

Optional: $3.00 per book for rush delivery ____________

TOTAL ____________

I understand that I may return any book for a full refund if not satisfied.

Name: ________________________________

Address: ________________________________

City: ________________________________

State, Zip: ________________________________

________Please send information about scheduling a MOVES Workshop in my area!

9494